D1274044

American Medical Association
Physicians dedicated to the health of America

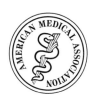

The Practical Guide to
Range of Motion Assessment

Assessment *First Edition*

John J. Gerhardt, MD

Linda Cocchiarella, MD, MSc

Randall D. Lea, MD

The Practical Guide to
Range of Motion Assessment
First Edition

Internet address: www.ama-assn.org

This book is for informational purposes only. It is not intended to
constitute legal or financial advice. If legal, financial, or other
professional advice is required, the services of a competent professional
should be sought.

Additional copies of this book may be ordered by calling 800 621-8335.
Mention product number OP120902.

ISBN 1-57947-263-X

BP90:02-P-0035:06/02

This practical guide is dedicated to all those who are striving to present objective, measured data as part of an evidence-based approach to the evaluation and reporting of impairment and disability.

John Gerhardt, MD

Linda Cocchiarella, MD, MSc

Randall Lea, MD

Measurement of joint range of motion (ROM) is important to the field of impairment rating and disability evaluation for a number of reasons. Joint ROM along with strength, endurance, coordination, and sensation are among the essential determinants of musculoskeletal function. The physician who seeks to diagnose or treat such limitations of musculoskeletal function must be able to accurately and objectively evaluate and record joint ROM. Also, there is a strong need for simplification and standardization to facilitate communication among practitioners and researchers. This could be potentially accomplished by using a universal method and language of measurement and recording with numbers.

Through ROM measurement, physicians and other health care examiners can identify and properly record loss of function in terms of joint ROM, for diagnosis, documenting treatment goals and response. It is sometimes essential for meeting statutory and legal requirements for impairment rating and disability determination. With the publication of *The Practical Guide to Range of Motion Assessment*, the American Medical Association and the authors have taken an important step toward standardizing measurement of joint motion in an accessible publication for health care examiners.

The approach discussed in *The Practical Guide to Range of Motion Assessment*, is based upon the Neutral-Zero Method of measurement, which was adopted by the American Academy of Orthopaedic Surgeons, the American Society for Surgery of the Hand and other international associations interested in a standardized approach to ROM measurement. Standardized approaches to recording ROM methods, such as the SFTR Recording Method, are also discussed in this manual, and have been widely used in Europe for decades.

The Practical Guide to Range of Motion Assessment builds upon the work of a number of individuals and associations who have been longstanding proponents for the adoption of a simplified and uniform approach to ROM measurement that employs a universally accepted methodology, terminology, and recording. Among them, the work of John J. Gerhardt has appeared previously in the national and international literature, and was succinctly presented in his *Documentation of Joint Motion*, 4th Edition (2) in 1994. It remained a well kept secret among examiners until recently, and is only now receiving the attention it deserves (3).

Although the American Medical Association *Guides to the Evaluation of Permanent Impairment* (AMA *Guides,* 4th Edition)(4) included some standardization to ROM measurement, specific techniques and applications were not clearly defined. The AMA *Guides* 5th Edition, (5) and *Master the Guides*-5th Edition *(6)* provided a standardized approach to range of motion measurements, but because of their scope and content, could not lend themselves to full descriptions and illustrations of the array of ROM measurement techniques and recording, which are of critical importance to the health care examiner. Consequently, the authors of *The Practical Guide to Range of Motion Assessment* filled this void through a thoughtful, detailed, and illustrated description of a standardized approach to ROM measurement and recording. This work should serve as a useful companion reference not only to the AMA *Guides,* but for users of other disability systems who seek to improve their measurement accuracy and reliability when evaluating physical impairments of the spine and extremities.

The measurement and recording system discussed in this book is both straightforward and elegant. This book is comprised of two parts. Part 1 deals with the principles and standardized approach to the assessment of joint ROM according to the Neutral Zero Recording and SFTR Documentation System. The use of goniometers and inclinometers, and calibration and stabilization procedures applicable to these devices are covered here. Part 2 deals with measurement procedures and techniques for specific joints of the body, regionally divided into the spine, upper, and lower extremities. Measurement and recording techniques for key joints of interest are described and illustrated in appreciable detail. The reader will find that this format lends itself equally well to self-directed instruction and future reference and review.

In summary, *The Practical Guide to Range of Motion Assessment* directs the field of impairment and disability rating toward further standardization of ROM measurement. Examiners who seek to apply and perfect their skills in ROM measurement and all parties who seek greater reproducibility and accuracy will benefit from use of this *Practical Guide.*

Robert D. Rondinelli, MD, PhD
Professor & Chairman
Department of Rehabilitation Medicine
University of Kansas Medical Center
Kansas City, KS 66160-7306

REFERENCES

1. American Academy of Orthopaedic Surgeons, Committee for the Study of Joint Motion. *Joint Motion: Method of Measuring and Recording*, Chicago. The American Academy of Orthopaedic Surgeons, 1965.

2. Gerhardt JJ. *Documentation of Joint Motion, International Standard Neutral-Zero Measuring, S.F.T.R. Recording and Application of Goniometers, Inclinometers and Calipers,* 4th Edition. Portland: ISOMED, Inc., 1994.

3. Gerhardt JJ, Rondinelli RD. Goniometric techniques for range-of-motion assessment. In: Rondinelli RD, Katz RT (eds.) *Disability Evaluation. Phys Med Rehabil Clin N Am* 12(3):507-27, 2001.

4. American Medical Association. *Guides to the Evaluation of Permanent Impairment,* 4th Edition. Eds Doege T, Houston T. Chicago: American Medical Association, 1993.

5. American Medical Association. *Guides to the Evaluation of Permanent Impairment,* 5th Edition. Eds Cocchiarella L, Andersson G. Chicago: American Medical Association, 2001.

6. Cocchiarella L, Lord SJ. *Master the AMA Guides 5th: A Medical and Legal Transition to the Guides to the Evaluation of Permanent Impairment,* 5th Edition, Chicago: American Medical Association, 2001.

7. Lea RD, Gerhardt JJ. Current Concepts Review, Range-of-Motion Measurements. *JBJS* 77-A, no. 5, 784-798, 1995.

The American Medical Association's (AMA's) new book *The Practical Guide to Range of Motion Assessment* shows users how to reproducibly and accurately measure range of motion (ROM). This book will be a welcome addition to users of the AMA *Guides to the Evaluation of Permanent Impairment (Guides)*, since it provides additional instruction, beyond the AMA *Guides*, of how to measure ROM, in a systematic format for more accurate evaluation of impairment.

Although range of motion measurements can provide extremely valuable information about physical functions, their use has been limited, partly due to criticism regarding limited reproducibility. Problems with reproducibility have been noted among examiners and by the same examiner and examinee on different occasions. This is understandable considering the fact that there is no standardized approach to measurements of range of motion, there are no standardized features of instruments and the variability of instruments and their application does not lend itself to consistent readings or comparability. Without standardization neither consistent nor reproducible measurements of range of motion can be achieved.

Although some variability is inevitable due to the dynamic nature of the human body and its condition, variability can be greatly reduced with appropriate instrumentation, training of examiners, consistent measurement techniques, suitable warm-up exercises and accurate recording of measurements. This book provides the needed instruction to limit these potential sources of variability and error.

The Practical Guide uses pictures, which truly "speak a thousand words" to teach the user in a step by step fashion the proper method to obtain and record ROM measurements for greater reproducibility and accuracy.

This book can be used either as a companion to the AMA *Guides*, or independently for those interested in ROM techniques. It will be especially useful to all health professionals: physicians, physical and occupational therapists, nurses, and nurse practitioners and others who seek to understand and evaluate ROM. It will also be helpful to researchers for studies to establish normative data.

Key features of *The Practical Guide to Range of Motion Assessment:*

- Presentation of the modified Neutral Zero Measuring Method

- Detailed description of the standardized SFTR Numerical Documentation System

- Discussion of instrumentation and standardized features of instruments

- Details on standardized warm-up exercises prior to taking measurements

- Standardized anatomical landmarks and terminology

- Standardized gravity-related starting -0- positions

- Background on the importance of proper positioning of the examinee, the evaluator, and needed stabilization for the body, the extremities and instrumentation

- Application of standardized measuring techniques

- An overview of key variables, which affect ROM measurements, indicating which can be controlled by the examiner and examinee

- Illustrations and annotated photographs, presented in a step-by-step fashion, indicating how ROM measurements are taken and recorded

The Practical Guide is suitable for individuals with training in ROM measurement and those who need to learn the standardized techniques. Users will find it a welcome addition to their libraries for ensuring reproducible, consistent, and accurate data for the evaluation of impairment and disability.

John Gerhardt MD

Linda Cocchiarella MD, MSc

Randall Lea MD

Thank you to the following members of the AMA Press:

Anthony J. Frankos, Vice President, Business Products

Mary Lou White, Executive Director, Editorial

Jean Roberts, Director, Production and Manufacturing

Barry Bowlus, Senior Acquisitions Editor

Pat Lee, Technical Developmental Editor

Katharine Dvorak, Developmental Editor

Mary Albanese, Image Coordinator

Boon Ai Tan, Senior Production Coordinator

Rosalyn Carlton, Senior Production Coordinator

Ronnie Summers, Senior Print Coordinator

Reg Schmidt, Marketing Manager

Ted Grudzinski, Medical Photographer

David Arispe, Editorial Assistant

Also, thank you to Barbara Stratton, Fitness Instructor, and Herta McClenahan, Personal Trainer, for outlining and describing the standardized warm-up exercises.

Special Acknowledgment

Scientific progress results from understanding the work of many individuals who often have revolutionary ideas. A scientist selects the best ones, adds new ones, combines, modifies, and then builds upon them.

My gratitude goes to all who laid the groundwork that led to the evolution of the presented approach to objective measurements. I would like to acknowledge the pioneers who preceded me whose work has not been widely recognized before:

Margaret Moore, PhD, PT, who standardized application of the conventional goniometer, called attention to the need for uniform recording, and greatly improved the accuracy of measurements of joint motion;

Jules Rippstein, MD, who first attempted to standardize instrumentation for measuring range of motion by indicating gravity in his PLURIMETER System;

Carter Rowe, MD, Chairman of the American Academy of Orthopedic Surgeons Committee on joint measurements, who introduced me to the original and modified Neutral -0- Measuring Method of Cave and Roberts;

Otto Russe, MD, who recognized the advantages of the Neutral -0- Measuring Method and the numerical SFTR Documentation System and introduced both in Europe where they became a mandatory standard in several countries.

Johannes Schlaaff, MD, who developed and standardized his 360-degree Measuring Fan, and Finger Fan, and introduced a numerical recording system of joint motion in two planes and rotation.

John Gerhardt, MD

Personal Dedication

To my friends, mentors and loved ones, who have taught me the meaning of dedication, perseverance, integrity, teamwork, leadership and love: M and P Baubley, D and R Bennett, S Darnell, J Gerhardt, L Haley, E Katrakis, J Regna, M Robling, M Salour.

To my greatest teachers and dear family: J Cocchiarella, and M Cocchiarella.

To all injured workers, their employers, colleagues and families: may compassion and peace be yours.

Linda Cocchiarella, MD, MSc

Recognition

The American Academy of Disability Evaluating Physicians (AADEP) pursues research and education in the field of evaluation of impairment and disability, emphasizing objective, standardized measurements. For this, I would like to recognize their contribution to this new, developing field of medicine.

Randall Lea, MD

Principles of Standardized Range of Motion Measurement

chapter 1

Key Principles

Range of motion (ROM) is one of the primary tools used to assess musculoskeletal function.[1] Most impairment rating guides in the United States and abroad include some form of range of motion measurement as a basis for assigning impairment (eg, the American Medical Association's *Guides to the Evaluation of Permanent Impairment* [*Guides*],[2] the *Florida Guides*,[3] and the *Minnesota Guides*.[4] The purpose of introducing range of motion measurements into the *Guides* was to a) include an aspect of function that was not entirely accounted for by diagnosis alone; b) provide an objective measurement for an aspect of function that was not subject to opinion as diagnosis may be; and c) account for individual variability within a particular diagnosis. The Fifth Edition of the *Guides* provides greater detail on the measurement and interpretation of range of motion compared with earlier editions. However, it assumes the user has significant experience in range of motion determination. Unfortunately, formal instruction on range of motion measurement for most physicians is minimal. Moreover, measurement of range of motion is sometimes performed by other health care providers who may have had different training in range of motion measurements, adding additional variability to these measurements.

The purpose of this range of motion manual is to provide detailed instruction on a standardized methodology for measuring range of motion and, thus, enable physicians and other evaluators to obtain more reliable range of motion measurements by using the same standardized protocols, reference tables, and reporting methods.[5] Although the text and pictorial material are designed to enable the examiner to achieve a standardized and reproducible technique, it is not a substitute for a hands-on training program or practice under proper supervision.

Part 1 of this manual discusses the general principles of standardized range of motion measurement, and includes a discussion of instrumentation, positioning and stabilization of the body, warm-up exercises, and recording the measurements and evaluating factors that affect range of motion measurements. Some illustrations and photos appear as well.

Part 2 provides numerous instructions, illustrated diagrams, and photos enabling the examiner to achieve a standardized and reproducible technique for measuring range of motion in the most commonly measured body joints.

PRINCIPLES FOR MEASUREMENT OF RANGE OF MOTION

Range of motion measurements refer to the full range of movement in which a body part moves. Although range of motion is objectively measured, there are still a number of factors that can influence measurement accuracy. The measurement of joint range of motion may vary slightly among examiners due to "true variability" or normal physiologic changes within the body part; "subjective states" of the examinee, which can influence their effort; and "preventable variability" due to errors on the part of the examiner, the instrumentation, or its technical limitations.

Table 1-8 in Part 1 lists common factors and conditions that influence ROM. (See page 19.)

The measurement of compound and complex joint motions (eg, subtalar motion) can be difficult, as stabilizing adjacent body parts may be problematic.[6] Despite these limitations, range of motion is still considered to be one element of the clinical assessment that provides important information on aspects of muscle function. This manual seeks to decrease variability in range of motion measurements by alerting the evaluator to conditions that lead to variability and by providing a reproducible protocol for the measurement of range of motion. To obtain accurate ROM measurements, the evaluator must adhere to the following procedural principles:

1. Prepare the examinee psychologically and physically

2. Identify anatomical landmarks

3. Have the individual perform standardized warm-up exercises

4. Properly position and stabilize the body

5. Appropriately select, apply, and stabilize the instrumentation

6. Use the standardized Neutral Zero Measuring Method and proper measuring techniques

7. Accurately record measurements in the standardized numerical documentation of the SFTR system

8. Recognize and evaluate the importance of the factors affecting range of motion

1. Prepare the Examinee

The examinee should be prepared physically and psychologically so that maximal consistency and reproducibility of measurements can be achieved. To prepare the person physically, ask him or her to perform the standard warm-up exercises that are relevant for the indicated body part. Psychological preparation includes explanation of the reason for doing measurements, reassurance that the measurements should not cause pain or additional injury, description of the procedure, showing the instruments and demonstrating their functions, telling the examinee what is expected of him or her in regard to effort and cooperation, and actually demonstrating the desired range of motion to be measured. Ideally, this should minimize the person's apprehension and anxiety, and reduce possible errors in measurement.

2. Identify Anatomical Landmarks

The second principle requires accurate identification of the anatomical landmarks proximal and distal to the joint being measured. This is an absolute necessity so that consistent, subsequent measurements can be obtained. Inaccuracies in landmark identification have been found to result in significant variability when measuring range of motion of the spine as well as the peripheral joints.[35-38]

For example, in the spine, to find T1 palpate C7 (vertebra prominens) and count 1 level down. To find T12 palpate the lower scapular angle, which is the T8 level. Project a horizontal line to the spine and count 4 levels down.

To verify this level, palpate the 12th (floating) rib and follow it to the spine. The 2 marks should coincide and indicate the 12th spinal process. (See Figure 1-1)

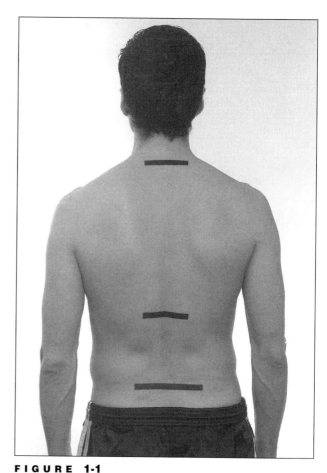

F I G U R E 1-1

Cervical spine anatomical landmarks: T1, T12, and S1, S2.

To find the landmark over the Sacrum, palpate the PSIS (posterior, superior, iliac spines), which are just caudal to the skin dimples that are usually clearly visible even in obese individuals. The PSIS are at the S2 level and should be horizontal. Place a skin mark or tape connecting the left and right PSIS. If they are not horizontal, it usually indicates either a true or apparent leg shortening. They should be level prior to taking ROM measurements. First, try the Thompson maneuver for 10 to 20 seconds to reestablish the proper relationship between the ilium and sacrum. See numbers 19 and 20 in the Descriptions of Warm-up Exercises on page 6. If this does not correct the tilt, use calibrated wooden blocks or heel lifts under the short leg until the PSIS are level.

When measuring hands and feet, see the illustrations for anatomical landmarks shown (Figures 1-2 and 1-3).

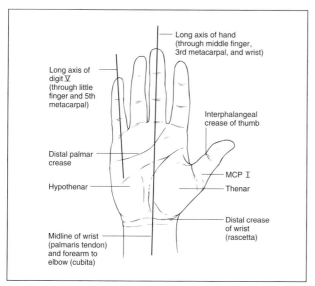

FIGURE 1-2

Anatomical landmarks of the hand: palmar view, right hand.

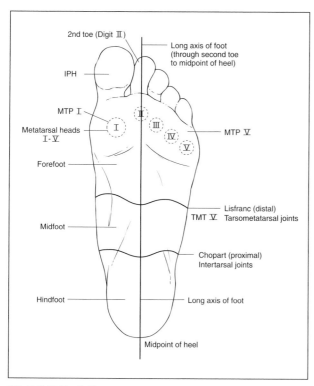

FIGURE 1-3

Anatomical landmarks of the foot: plantar view, left foot.

Other landmarks are discussed in Part 2.

3. Have the Individual Perform Standardized Warm-up Exercises

Warm-up exercises done prior to measurements of range of motion are very important because they can reduce the possibility of muscle strain, ligamentous sprain, or secondary injury and greatly increase accuracy, consistency, and reproducibility of the measurements.[5,32,58] However, for rating purposes, precautions should be taken to avoid discomfort.[58] Warm-up exercises should not be done if an individual came for an evaluation, but has not reached maximal medical improvement.

The following exercise list represents the minimum exercises needed to warm up the major muscles involved in stabilizing and moving joints. A selection of these exercises can be chosen for strictly regional measurements. See also warm-up exercises in Part 2, which are shown under the specific anatomical area to be measured.

Descriptions of Warm-up Exercises

Have the examinee perform these exercises slowly, at the individual's chosen pace. Discontinue the exercises if the individual develops pain. The examiner needs to adjust the type and difficulty of the exercises if the individual has had any recent injury, surgery, or joint replacement or a medical condition that would make exercising inadvisable.

1. Sit in a chair away from the backrest and march the legs in place, moving the arms in an alternating forward and backward motion, 8 times. Keep the elbows at the side of the body.

2. Continue marching with the legs, lift the extended arms sideways and overhead slowly two times; then extend both arms overhead and pull one down, then reverse, alternating arms (one arm up, and the other down) two times.

3. Continue marching with the legs, holding the extended arms in front of the body, then open the arms wide and pull back. Repeat 4 times.

4. Extend one leg on the floor with the knee straight, press the heel out with toes up toward the body, then bend the knee and place the foot flat close to the chair. Alternate right and left 4 times. Continue leg movements and add arm movements; reach out extending the elbows and pull back flexing the elbows. Repeat 4 times.

5. Place the legs in a wide straddle. March the legs and move the arms with the elbows flexed forward and back, alternating the left and right arms 4 times.

6. Roll the shoulders backward 2 times and then reverse 2 times.

7. Move the shoulders up, down, forward and backward 4 times.

8. Move the left arm up with the elbow bent over the head and bend the trunk slowly to the right 2 times. Next repeat the exercise with the right arm over the head, elbow bent and bend the trunk slowly to the left 2 times.

9. Place the right hand over the left shoulder and upper arm, then grab the right elbow with the left hand and pull to the left to stretch the right shoulder. Hold for a count of 4, then reverse to stretch the left shoulder.

10. Pull the stomach in, exhale, and round the back slowly. Hold this position for a count of 4, then straighten slowly to upright sitting position while inhaling, hold for a count of 2. Repeat 2 times.

11. Sit straight and bend sideways reaching the hand toward the floor two times right and left.

12. Sit straight with the knees together in front and gently turn the trunk and the head to the left 2 times and to the right 2 times.

13. Keep the heels on the floor and tap the toes up and down, alternating left and right, 8 times.

14. Tap the left toes with the heels on the floor and placed about 4 inches apart, 4 times, then rotate the foot in and out 4 times. Repeat with the right toes and foot.

15. Move the heels up and down together 8 times.

16. Lift and hold the left knee up with both hands, rotate the left ankle and foot clockwise 4 times, and then reverse 4 times. Lift and hold the right knee and rotate the right ankle and foot clockwise 4 times, then reverse 4 times.

17. Keep the elbows flexed at the side of the body with the forearms pointed forward. Then supinate and pronate the forearms (palms up, palms down) 4 times. Extend and flex the wrists (move the hands up and down from the wrist) 4 times. Move the wrists into radial and ulnar deviation (move them in and out) 4 times. Move the thumbs and fingers as if playing the piano up and down the keyboard, 4 times.

18. Start with the arms hanging straight at the side of the body, then while inhaling slowly, move the arms above the head. Next, while exhaling, move the arms slowly down. Repeat 2 times.

Do one of the two following alternatives of Thompson's corrective exercises (19 or 20).[58]

19. A1: Stand facing the back of the chair. Hold on to the back of the chair, keep the feet 1 foot apart and turn them 45° out. Next, spread the thighs while keeping the knees over the toes, and make 10 half-knee bends keeping the trunk as straight as possible.

20. A2: Sit straight on the edge of a chair, spread the thighs as wide as comfortably possible and turn the feet 45° out. Bend the trunk forward and down, rounding the back, so that the elbows are touching the inner side of the knees and the fingers are close to the floor. (Make sure that the knees are aligned over the toes.) Hold this position for 20 seconds and then return to the upright sitting position.

21. To stand up, keep the legs straddled, bring the feet close to the chair and stand up without bending the trunk forward. (Use your leg muscles and not your back muscles.)

22. An alternative technique for getting up from a chair follows. (The same technique may also be used for getting up from a bench or bed.) From a sitting position with the feet on the floor, place the arms behind the hips and push yourself forward to the edge of the chair without bending forward. Turn 90° on the chair to either the left or right side and hold on to the backrest of the chair. Have the knee closest to the chair flexed 90° and the foot on that side flat on the floor. Move the other leg backward with the knee almost at kneeling position and the weight on the bent toes. Straighten the knees and push yourself up into upright position.

4. Properly Position and Stabilize the Body

Practically speaking, joint motion can be measured in the standing, sitting, supine, prone, lateral decubitus position, or in some combination of these positions. Several factors, such as the type of measuring device or physical limitations of the examinee, can dictate the optimal position. For example, inclinometric measurement of cervical rotation must be done with the examinee in the supine position since inclinometers reference gravity. Horizontal movements in the sitting position would not show a change as the plane of movement with respect to gravity does not change. Positions maximizing examinee comfort may be helpful in determining the maximum range of motion an individual is able to obtain.[39-42] Finally, whatever position is utilized, stabilize and evaluate both the body and proximal part of the joint as instability secondary to positioning has been found to be a significant source of error by multiple investigators.[33,43-45,58,59]

5. Select, Apply, and Stabilize Instrumentation

The tools used to measure range of motion vary from simplistic visual estimation to complex optoelectronic systems.[25-28] Although complex systems may not be an absolute necessity, instrumentation has been shown to be more accurate than visual estimation in measuring range of motion.[29-32,33] The two main devices currently used to measure range of motion are goniometers and inclinometers. See Figure 1-4 and Figure 1-5. Their strengths and limitations are outlined in Table 1-1.

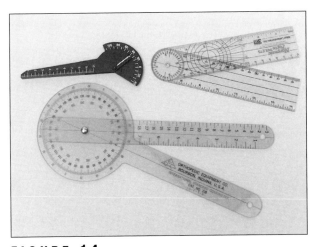

FIGURE 1-4

Examples of typical two-arm goniometers and finger goniometer.

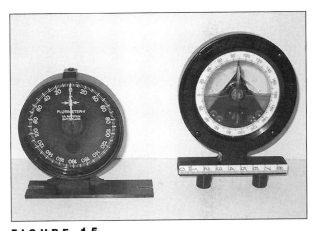

FIGURE 1-5

Examples of mechanical and fluid level inclinometers.

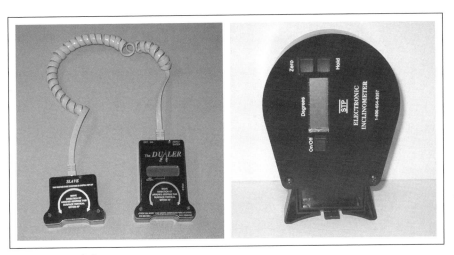

FIGURE 1-6

Examples of electronic inclinometers.

TABLE 1-1

Comparison of the Goniometer and Inclinometer

Feature	Goniometer	Inclinometer (Manual)	Inclinometer (Electronic)
Axis measurement	Only simple movements, not complex	All movements	All movements
Dependence on visual alignment	Total dependence	Partial dependence of alignment; all positions accurately measured due to automatic display of gravity	Partial dependence of alignment; requires calibration to gravity before each measurement
Accuracy	Subjective; visual assessment of starting position	Improved, due to automatic display of gravity and starting position referenced to gravity; accuracy dependent on ability to stabilize instrument on body	Improved; needs calibration to gravity before each measurement; accuracy dependent on ability to stabilize instrument on body
Reproducibility	Fair; relies on visual assessment	Improved; gravity already displayed, reproducibility depends on proper stabilization and training	Improved; gravity already displayed, reproducibility depends on proper stabilization and training
Ease of use	Fairly easy	Fairly easy	Easy when familiar with instrument
Measures compound spine motions	Inadequate	Adequate	Adequate
Individual positioning	Any position acceptable	Place inclinometer vertically for proper functioning; relies on gravity; adjust individual's position	Place inclinometer vertically for proper functioning; relies on gravity; adjust individual's position
Cost	Very inexpensive	Relatively inexpensive	Expensive

The two-arm goniometer is probably the most widely used instrument to measure joint motion. It consists of two arms, a stationary arm and a movable arm; a protractor with degrees from 0 to 180 or 0 to 360, which is attached to one arm. The two arms are linked with a central axis. The goniometer has significant limitations in that it cannot measure complex and compound motions such as those seen within the spine, forearm, or foot.[5,58] Goniometers require the user to visually align the arms with the components of the joint and/or the anatomical landmarks, which can be difficult to identify. Thus, it is difficult to know if the goniometer is being placed at the same starting positions on successive measurements, which can reduce reproducibility[5,58] (Figure 1-7, Figure 1-8). Goniometers also require the examiner to have greater dexterity and precision as two hands are used simultaneously: one hand keeps one goniometer arm stationary while the other hand moves the other moveable goniometer arm with the body part. The advantages of the two-armed goniometers are that they can be used in any position (upright, supine, and so on) and are portable and inexpensive.[33]

Inclinometers may also be used to measure joint motion. These devices, if properly designed, read angle position relative to gravity or to a set neutral -0- position. The primary advantage of this type of device is that it enables the examiner to identify the same starting position on successive measurements. That is, since gravity does not change, the starting position can be consistently identified and repeated. All inclinometers function on the principle of gravity and must be held vertically to function properly. The position of the examinee has to be adjusted accordingly. For example, he or she must be in the supine position when cervical rotation is being measured.

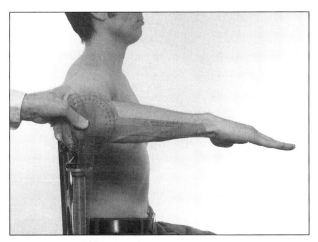

FIGURE 1-7

Goniometer used for measurement of shoulder rotation is not accurate because the position of the stationary arm has been visually assessed and is not quite in vertical position.

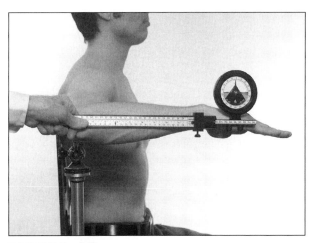

FIGURE 1-8

Inclinometer with attached extender indicates gravity and therefore yields a consistent, measured starting position.

Inclinometers may be mechanical or electronic. The mechanical inclinometers are based upon a fluid level or a weighted pendulum. In the fluid-type inclinometers, the fluid level indicates the horizontal position. Errors of reading may be caused by not specifying whether the degrees are read at the upper or lower meniscus of the fluid level. The evaluator needs to choose to read measurements at either the upper or lower meniscus and use this method consistently. The pendulum-weighted inclinometer has a -0- starting position indicated by the weighted needle or pendulum. It is important that the examiner stand perpendicular to the dial of the inclinometer to avoid reading errors caused by parallax.[58]

There are also electronic inclinometers with specially programmed software and recording systems that enable the electronic storage of a neutral -0- position in two different positions. This feature allows for spinal range of motion measurement using only one inclinometer. However, when such single inclinometric techniques are used, the movement of one inclinometer from one -0- position to the other can be accompanied by examinee movement and make the storage of the first -0- position obsolete. When two inclinometers are on each end of the measured segment, continual electronic observation and measurement of the positions of both inclinometers can adjust for minor movements of the individual. Unfortunately, such complex electronic systems remain relatively expensive. The two inclinometer technique can be effectively applied with two mechanical inclinometers.

The Fifth Edition of the *Guides to the Evaluation of Permanent Impairment* requires that an inclinometer be used for spine range of motion measurement. Because spinal motion is both compound and complex, identification of movement within a single spine region necessitates simultaneous measurements at both ends of the measured segment and subsequent mathematical subtraction of the motion segment below the segment of interest. Using the goniometer along multiple positions of the spine with only visual guidance is too error prone and, therefore, the inclinometer is required for more accurate readings.[33] This manual provides instructions for using the inclinometer when measuring spinal range of motion, and also gives a description for measuring range of motion of all other joints using a properly designed inclinometer.

Inclinometric measurement of the large joints of the extremities require the use of an extender attached to the inclinometer to allow proper alignment with the distal component of the joint being measured.[5,34,58] Application of the inclinometer on the distal part of large joints is often inaccurate because of variations in shape of the extremities, adiposity, or edema.[58] The extender effectively converts the inclinometer into a single-arm goniometer with the advantage of having a built-in indicator of gravity, which allows superior accuracy and reproducibility of measurements. If the examiner chooses to use the goniometer for measuring range of motion of the extremities, he or she should also refer to instructions provided in the Fifth Edition of the *Guides*. However, he or she should be aware of the disadvantages and errors in using two-arm goniometers that are related to visual assessment of starting positions.

Some instruments cannot be adequately stabilized, because of problems in their design. For example, a large inclinometer with a flat base cannot be properly stabilized on the spine because the flat base will toggle and shift on the spinous processes, causing errors of up to 20°.[58] Inclinometers with two rigid rather than adjustable protrusions can be applied across two spinous processes; however, the spinous processes distract in flexion and approximate in extension, which may cause the rigid protrusion to fall into the interspinous spaces, resulting in potential errors. An inclinometer with adjustable protrusions or legs should allow for adjustments due to individual anatomical differences, and enable the device to be stabilized on one level even when the adjacent spinous process moves. Such adjustable legs can also be applied to the appropriate landmark on small joints such as on the phalanges between the deformed joints with rheumatoid arthritis.[5,58]

Various goniometric designs have also been developed to assist with the differing application and stabilization requirements and ease of application. (eg, Pluri-dig goniometer for the digits and hand).[5,34,58]

How to Calibrate Mechanical and Electronic Inclinometers

Mechanical inclinometers that are precalibrated such as the Plurimeter,[5,34] Uni-level, or Bi-level[58] inclinometers, show gravity automatically. They can be set to horizontal gravity -0- or vertical gravity -0- position simply by holding the base approximately horizontal or vertical and turning the dial until a distinct click is felt and heard at the zero mark (Figures 1-9 a–d). The "0" on the dial indicates, then, the true horizontal or vertical position of the base of the inclinometer. Electronic inclinometers need to be calibrated before each measurement and the zero button must be held down until the inclinometer is stabilized in the zero starting position. It is necessary to have an adequate carpenter's level or true vertical and horizontal surfaces against which to calibrate.

To find the horizontal gravity -0- position for an inclinometer, hold the inclinometer against the horizontal surface of the carpenter's level or another true horizontal surface, and push and hold the zero out button down. To find the vertical gravity -0- position, hold the inclinometer against the vertical surface of the carpenter's level or another true vertical surface, and push and hold the zero out button down. See Figures 1-9c and 1-9e.

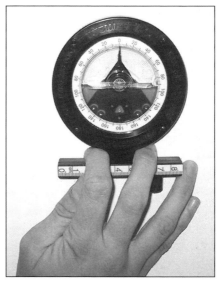

FIGURE 1-9a

The base of the precalibrated mechanical inclinometer is held approximately horizontal. To set, the dial is rotated and clicks into 0 position.

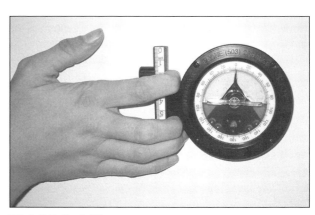

FIGURE 1-9b

The base of the precalibrated mechanical inclinometer is held approximately vertical. To set, the dial is rotated and clicks into 0 position.

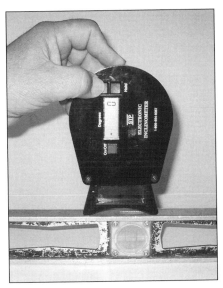

FIGURE 1-9c

Calibration of an electronic inclinometer in horizontal -0-gravity position on a carpenter's level placed horizontally.

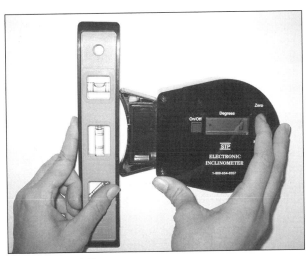

FIGURE 1-9e

Calibration of an electronic goniometer in vertical gravity zero position on a carpenter's level held vertically.

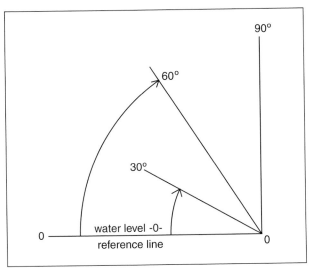

FIGURE 1-9d

Angle illustration showing horizontal reference 0.

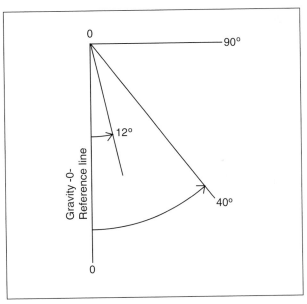

FIGURE 1-9f

Angle illustration showing vertical reference 0.

6. Use the Standardized Neutral Zero Measuring Method and Proper Measuring Techniques

A standardized measuring method, the Neutral Zero Measuring Method, became the method of preference in 1969 for describing range of motion. It was introduced by Cave and Roberts in 1935 to facilitate standardized measurements and communications, and then reintroduced in a modified version by the American Academy of Orthopedic Surgeons in the 1960s.[5,46,47]

The Neutral Zero Method defines the starting positions from the so-called anatomical position of the body: upright position, feet facing forward, arms at the side of the body, palms facing anteriorly (forward) (see Figures 1-10 a–d). If the individual changes position from the upright to sitting, supine, or prone position, the starting positions are always related back to the upright vertical position. This assures that the standardized, standing, neutral -0- starting position is consistent regardless of the individual's position and, thus, enhances consistency and reproducibility.

Once the neutral -0- position has been obtained, measurement can begin. Although opinions vary as to whether range of motion measurements should be determined more than once for accuracy, most references, including the *Guides*, suggest either using the greatest ROM measurement, from a series of reproducible measurements, or averaging several reproducible measurements. In general, unless some acute condition is present, multiple measurements are preferable to a single determination as reliability usually requires some level of repeatability.[2,58,59]

The evaluator must assess whether to measure active or passive range of motion. *Active* range of motion refers to a measurement made based upon the examinee moving the body part through its full range of motion without assistance or applying external force. With active range of motion, the individual is requested to move the particular body part to the maximum possible range even if some discomfort or mild pain ensues. The *Guides* requires active motion measurements for all determinations except supine straight-leg raising, which is a validity test. Active range of motion is allegedly more consistent than passive motion determinations and injury to the individual is unlikely as no external force is being applied. It may also be a better indicator of the range of motion used by the individual for normal activities of daily living and function.[48-57]

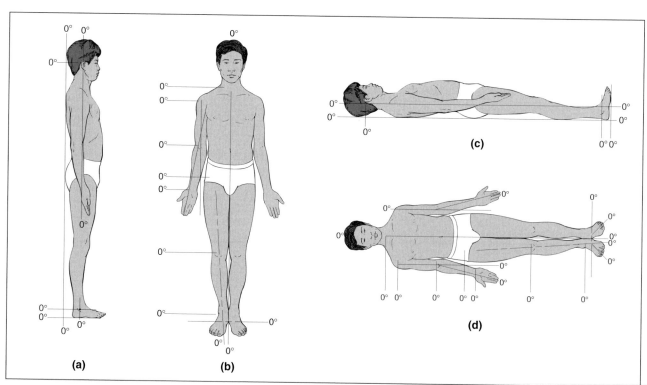

FIGURE 1-10

Four views of Neutral Zero Measuring Method: **(a)** standing: side view, **(b)** standing: front view, **(c)** laying: side view, **(d)** laying: on back

Adapted from Cocchiarella L, Andersson BJ, *Guides to the Evaluation of Permanent Impairment,* Fifth Edition, 2001, page 594.

The primary disadvantage of active range of motion is that it is more strongly influenced by individual subjective factors such as pain, effort, motivation, and attitude. Because active range of motion is significantly dependent on effort, the *Guides* recommends that multiple measurements be taken and only measurements within a specific reproducible range be considered reliable enough for rating purposes.

Passive range of motion measurements are taken when the examiner moves the examinee's body part through the maximum range of motion obtainable for that individual's specific condition. Passive range of motion may exceed active range of motion if the evaluator applies additional pressure to determine the inherent end point of motion. In such instances, passive range of motion may actually be a more accurate indicator of the actual motion possible. Disadvantages of the passive range of motion include measurement differences due to variation in the amount of external force applied by the examiner and the possibility that the passive forces applied by the examiner could possibly cause additional injury.[58] (This manual refers only to active range of motion measurements as suggested by the *Guides*.)

Table 1-2 outlines and defines the possible joint motions for the major body parts, and notes the plane in which they are recorded. Figure 1-11 illustrates these planes of movement and measurement.

T A B L E 1-2

Joint Motions, Recorded Planes of Movement, and Relevant Body Parts

Joint Motion	Definition	Plane Recorded	Spine	Upper Extremity	Lower Extremity
Extension	Bending the spine backwards; in the joint extremities, straightening	S	X	X	X
Flexion	Bending the spine forward; in extremities, bending the distal part of the joint toward the proximal part	S	X	X	X
Abduction	Motion away from the midline	F		X	X
Adduction	Motion toward the midline	F		X	X
Eversion	Hindfoot and midfoot move away from the body	F			X
Inversion	Hindfoot and midfoot move toward the body	F			X
Rotation of the Spine	Circular arc around a central body axis	R	X		
Left Rotation of the Spine	Left shoulder moves backward and right shoulder moves forward	R	X		
Right Rotation of the Spine	Right shoulder moves backward and left shoulder moves forward	R	X		
External Rotation of Extremities	Rotation away from the midline of the body	R		X	X
Internal Rotation of Extremities	Rotation toward the midline of the body	R		X	X
Supination	Rotary movement of extremity away from the midline so palm is up or plantar surface is toward the midline	R		X	X
Pronation	Rotary movement of extremity toward the midline so palm is down or plantar surface is toward outward	R		X	X

Key: S = sagittal, F = frontal, R = rotation

7. Accurately Record Measurements in the Numerical SFTR System

Measurements of range of motion are recorded in different formats such as descriptive, numerical, or a combination of both. This hinders efficient communication, retrieval of data, and meaningful comparisons. In an appendix of the Fifth Edition of the *Guides* the SFTR system was introduced. The SFTR system is one method for numerical recording of range of motion measurements. The SFTR acronym stands for the basic planes through which motion can occur. *S* represents the sagittal plane, which divides the body into the left and right halves. Planes parallel to this plane are also called sagittal planes. *F* represents the frontal plane, which divides the body into anterior and posterior halves and is perpendicular to the sagittal plane. Planes parallel to this plane are also called frontal planes.

T indicates the transverse plane, which divides the body into upper and lower segments at the center of gravity and is perpendicular to both the sagittal and frontal planes. Planes parallel to this plane transecting other parts of the body are also called transverse planes. The term "horizontal plane" should not be used to avoid confusion. In an upright position, the transverse plane is horizontal, but in a supine position the transverse plane is vertical. The individual has to be positioned supine or in lateral recumbent position if measurements in the transverse plane are required. *R* represents rotation and was added to facilitate recording of rotatory movements. For rotations, the term "axial plane" or "transaxial plane" is often used, but this refers to the transverse plane in the spine only and not to the extremities, in which rotations can take place in any of the 3 basic planes.[58,59]

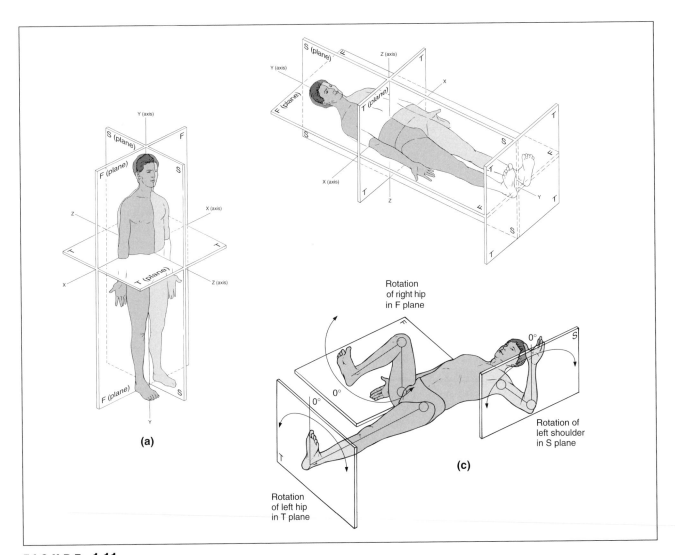

FIGURE 1-11

The three basic planes; sagittal, frontal, and transverse and cardinal axes x, y, and z in upright **(a)** and supine **(b)** positions. **(c)** Rotation can occur in any of the three basic planes.

Adapted from Cocchiarella L, Andersson BJ, *Guides to the Evaluation of Permanent Impairment*, Fifth Edition, 2001, page 402.

The SFTR system enables the user to standardize the recording of range of motion measurements. Motion is recorded with a letter designating the plane of motion or rotation, followed by three numbers with the starting position always in the middle. This figure shows an example of measuring and properly recording left and right lateral bending of the lumbar spine (Figure 1-12). Positions of ankylosis are recorded with one letter and two numbers. The degree of ankylosis and the 0 reference number are on either the left or right of the number. If the ankylosis is in extension, abduction, or external rotation, or in the spine, lateral bending to the left and left rotation, the number will be on the left side of 0. If the ankylosis is in flexion, adduction, or internal rotation, or in the spine right lateral

bending and right rotation, the number should be recorded to the right of 0. Using three numbers in a particular sequence reveals the motion, and follows the same format as measurement with the Neutral Zero Method, with the zero clearly identified as the starting position. In pathologic conditions in which the starting position is different from zero, the actual starting position is recorded in the middle rather than using 0. A middle number different from zero automatically indicates a pathologic limitation of motion. Additionally, if ankylosis is present, it is immediately recognized by the recording of two numbers only. The direction and range in which the ankylosis is present is readily identified depending on whether the zero is the first or second number. See Tables 1-3 through 1-6.

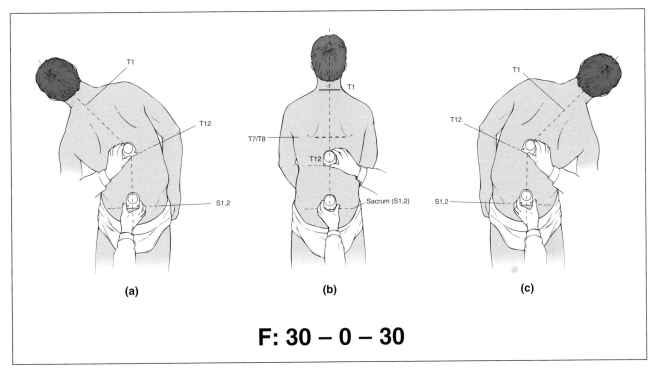

(a)   (b)   (c)

F: 30 – 0 – 30

FIGURE 1-12

Proper measurement and recording of **(a)** left lateral bending, **(b)** neutral -0- starting position and **(c)** right lateral bending of the lumbar spine. F: 30 -0- 30.

Adapted from Cocchiarella L, Andersson BJ, *Guides to the Evaluation of Permanent Impairment,* Fifth Edition, 2001, page 408.

TABLE 1-3

Example of the SFTR Recordings of Full, Limited, and Restricted Motion and Ankylosis of the Wrist in the Sagittal Plane (Extension and Flexion)

Motions and Ankyloses	SFTR Recording
1 NEUTRAL POSITION 0°	S: -0-
2 60° 0° EXTENSION 60° FLEXION 45° 45°	S:60-0-45
3 35° 10° 0° EXTENSION BETWEEN 35° AND 10°	S:35-10-0
4 30° 0° EXTENSION BETWEEN 30° AND 0°	S:30-0-0
5 0° FLEXION BETWEEN 0° AND 25° 25°	S:0-0-25
6 0° FLEXION BETWEEN 20° AND 50° 20° 50°	S:0-20-50
7 35° 0° ANKYLOSIS IN 35° EXTENSION	S:35-0
8 0° ANKYLOSIS IN 15° FLEXION 15°	S:0-15

Adapted from Gerhardt, JJ, *Documentation of Joint Motion: International Standard Neutral-Zero Measuring, S.F.T.R. Recording, Application of Goniometers, Inclinometers and Calipers,* Fourth Edition, 1994, page 8.

TABLE 1-4

Example of the SFTR Recordings of Full, Limited, and Restricted Motion and Ankylosis of the Elbow in the Sagittal Plane (Extension and Flexion)

Measured Motion of the Elbow	SFTR Recordings
Normal motion	S: 0 -0- 150
0 extension and flexion of 140°	S: 0 -0- 140
Hyperextension of 15°, flexion of 140°	S: 15 -0- 140
Flexion contracture of 30°, extension lag of 30° with further flexion to 90°	S: 0-30-90
Ankylosis in functional position of 80° of flexion	S: 0-80
Ankylosis in 15° of hyperextension	S: 15-0
Ankylosis in 20° of flexion	S: 0-20

S = sagittal plane

TABLE 1-5

Example of the SFTR Recordings of Full, Limited, and Restricted Motion and Ankylosis of the Ankle in the Sagittal Plane (Extension and Flexion) and the Frontal Plane (Valgus and Varus)

Measured Motion of the Ankle	SFTR Recordings
Normal motion	S: 20 -0- 45
Extension (dorsiflexion) of 10°, flexion (plantar flexion) of 20°	S: 10 -0- 20
Valgus of the calcaneus of 10° and Varus of the calcaneus of 20°	FC: 10 -0- 20
Ankylosis of the ankle in 20° of valgus	F: 20-0
Ankylosis of the ankle in 15° of varus	F: 0-15

S = sagittal plane, FC = calcaneus (frontal plane), F = frontal plane

TABLE 1-6

Example of the SFTR Recordings of Full, Limited, and Restricted Motion and Ankylosis of the Knee in the Sagittal Plane (Extension and Flexion) and the Frontal Plane (Valgus and Varus)

Measured Motion of the Knee	SFTR Recordings
Normal motion	S: 0 -0- 135
Hyperextension (back knee) of 15° and flexion of 135°	S: 15 -0- 135
Extension lag of 15° and flexion of 90°	S: 0-15-90
Ankylosis in 20° of flexion	S: 0-20
Ankylosis in neutral -0- starting position	S: 0-0
neutral -0- starting position in the frontal plane	F: 0 -0- 0
Unstable knee with passive motion from 5° of valgus to 10° of varus	F(p): 5 -0- 10
Ankylosis in valgus of 5°	F: 5-0
Ankylosis in varus of 15°	F: 0-15

S = sagittal plane, F = frontal plane, F(p) = passive motion in the frontal plane

For recording: (p) = passive motion, (a) = active motion

The planes and sequences of recording normal measurements are presented in Table 1-7.

T A B L E 1-7

Sequence of Recording Measurements in the SFTR System

Plane	First (to the left of 0°)	Neutral-0° (starting)	Last (to the right of 0°)
Sagittal (S)	Extension	-0-	Flexion
Frontal (F)	Abduction	-0-	Adduction
	Radial deviation	-0-	Ulnar deviation
	Elevation	-0-	Depression
	Valgus	-0-	Varus
	Eversion of hindfoot and midfoot	-0-	Inversion of hindfoot and midfoot
	Side bending of head and spine to the left	-0-	Side bending of head and spine to the right
Transverse (T)	Horizontal extension	-0-	Horizontal flexion
	Horizontal abduction	-0-	Horizontal adduction
	Retraction	-0-	Protraction
Rotation (R)	External rotation	-0-	Internal rotation
	Supination of forearm and forefoot	-0-	Pronation of forearm and forefoot
	External torsion	-0-	Internal torsion
	Rotation of head and spine to the left	-0-	Rotation of head and spine to the right

Adapted from Gerhardt, JJ, *Documentation of Joint Motion: International Standard Neutral-Zero Measuring, S.F.T.R. Recording, Application of Goniometers, Inclinometers and Calipers,* Fourth Edition, 1994, page 7.

8. Recognize and Evaluate the Importance of the Factors Affecting Range of Motion

The examiner may wish to discuss with the examinee any of the factors listed in Table 1-8, which affect ROM measurements.

TABLE 1-8

Factors and Conditions Associated with Range of Motion (ROM) Changes

I. Objective Factors

Demographic
- **Age.** ROM on some joints typically decreases with age.[7-20]
- **Sex.**[9, 13, 21-23]
- **Occupation.** ROM is greater in less sedentary positions.[24]

Injuries to Main or Associated Structures
- **Skin and connective tissue.** Injury, such as scars, contractures, laxity, swelling, or edema can cause limitation of motion.
- **Bone injury or disorders.** Fractures, angulations, shortening, displacements, compression, kyphosis, scoliosis, osteoporosis, bone replacement, osteotomy, laminectomy, plasticectomy, fusion, and other surgical interventions.
- **Joint.** Loss of joint play, degenerative joint disease, arthritis, subluxation, dislocation, fracture, contracture, bursitis, contusion, ankylosis, dysarticulation, and replacement (total or partial).
- **Ligament.** Laxity, sprain, tear, and others.
- **Muscle.** Spasticity, rigidity, spasm, changes in tone, trigger points, hypertrophy, atrophy, weakness, fatigue, strain, tear.
- **Nervous system.** Impaired motor or sensory function (eg, paresis, weakness, dysesthesia, paresthesia, astereognosis, altered position sense, vibration, nerve compression, stretch, neuropathy, and movement disorders such as tremor, athetosis, akinesis, bradykinesis, asynergism, gait abnormalities, and posture abnormalities).

External Influences[5]
- **Medication.** Especially when the medication affects muscle relaxation, inflammation, and pain. Note the time relevant medications were taken with respect to the medical evaluation.
- **Time of day.** Record the time measurements were taken and note conditions especially associated with time-related ROM changes (eg, arthritis).
- **Therapy.** Heat, cold, exercises, biofeedback.
- **Activity.** Activity will improve ROM.

II. Subjective Influences

- **Fatigue.** Usually results in decreased ROM.
- **Attitude.**
- **Pain.** Evaluate and record pain and the associated painful condition.
- **Emotional status.** Emotional stress, tension, depression may affect muscle flexibility and ROM.

III. Examiner Variability

- **Proper position and stabilization of the body.**
- **Selection, application, and stabilization of the instrumentation.**
- **Measuring techniques** (eg, warm-up exercises, number of repetitions, active vs passive movement).
- **Method of recording.**
- **Recognition and weighing of factors that affect ROM** (listed above).

How to Avoid Common Errors

1. Properly prepare the examinee (see page 4) and encourage his or her cooperation.

2. Identify anatomical landmarks correctly.

3. Perform the standardized warm-up exercises with the examinee before taking measurements.

4. Properly calibrate inclinometers that do not indicate gravity to horizontal or vertical gravity -0- position. Make certain that the objects that you are calibrating against have true vertical and horizontal surfaces. Digital displays do not indicate gravity.

5. Choose gravity-related starting positions and measure them with inclinometers. Never use visual assessment or guess by the "rule of thumb."

6. Properly position and stabilize the examinee and/or proximal component of the joint.

7. Set the inclinometer to vertical or horizontal gravity -0- position and stabilize it on the body and or distal component of the measured joint. In large joints, properly align the extender arm with the long axes of joint components. Ascertain that the inclinometer is stabilized on a single level on the spine. Avoid concomitant movements in other planes during measurements.

8. Stretch the skin when stabilizing inclinometers on loose skin overlying bone, such as on the scalp or forehead to avoid shifting of the inclinometer with the skin on the underlying bone. In general, do not stabilize the inclinometer on soft tissue.

9. Do not use Velcro to fasten inclinometers to the body except for dynamic measurements.

10. Read degrees indicated by mechanical inclinometers by facing the dial straight to avoid errors caused by parallax and use the upper or lower meniscus for reading fluid-type inclinometers consistently.

11. Record the planes of motion: sagittal (S), frontal (F), transverse (T), and rotation (R).

12. Become familiar with the instrument that you are using and know its technical limitations. (Call the manufacturer as necessary.) Learn correct measuring techniques before attempting measurements for rating purposes.

REFERENCES

1. Gerhardt JJ, Rondinelli RD. Goniometric techniques for range-of-motion assessment. *Phys Med Rehabil Clin North Am.* 2001;12:507-527.

2. Cocchiarella L, Andersson G. *Guides to the Evaluation of Permanent Impairment.* 5th ed. Chicago, Ill: AMA Press; 2000.

3. *Florida Uniform Permanent Impairment Rating Schedule.* Florida Worker's Compensation Institute, Inc., Call Box 200, Tallahassee, FL 32302-0200; 1996.

4. *Minnesota Guides.* TK

5. Gerhardt JJ. *Documentation of Joint Motion.* 4th ed. Portland, Ore: Isomed; 1994.

6. Mann RA. Principles of examination of the foot and ankle. In: Mann RA, ed. *Surgery of the Foot.* 5th ed. St Louis, MO: Mosby; 1986:31-49.

7. Buckwalter JA, Woo SL, Goldberg VM, Hadley EC, Booth F, Oegema TR, Eyre DR. Soft-tissue aging and musculoskeletal function. *J Bone Joint Surg Am.* 1993; 75:1533-1548.

8. Dopf CA, Mandel SS, Geiger DF, Mayer PJ. Analysis of spine motion variability using a computerized goniometer compared to physical examination: a prospective clinical study. *Spine.* 1994;19:586-595.

9. Dvorak J, Antinnes JA, Panjabi N, Loustalot D, Bonomo M. Age and gender related normal motion of the cervical spine. *Spine.* 1992;17(10 suppl):S393-398.

10. Einkauf DK, Gohdes ML, Jensen GM, Jewell MJ. Changes in spinal mobility with increasing age in women. *Phys Ther.* 1987;67:370-375.

11. Ferlic D. The range of motion of the "normal" cervical spine. *Bull Johns Hopkins Hosp.* 1962;110:59-65.

12. Fitzgerald GK, Wynveen KJ, Rheault W, Rothschild B. Objective assessment with establishment of normal values for lumbar spinal range of motion. *Phys Ther.* 1983;63: 1776-1781.

13. Hayashi H, Okada K, Hamada M, Tada K, Ueno R. Etiologic factors of myelopathy: a radiographic evaluation of the aging changes in the cervical spine. *Clin Orthop.* 1987;214:200-209.

14. Lind B, Sihlbom H, Nordwall A, Malchau H. Normal range of motion of the cervical spine. *Arch Phys Med Rehabil.* 1989;70:692-695.

15. Loebl WY. Measurement of spinal posture and range of spinal movement. *Ann Phys Med.* 1967;9:103-110.

16. Moll JM, Wright V. Normal range of spinal mobility: an objective clinical study. *Ann Rheum Dis.* 1971;30:381-386.

17. Moll JM, Liyanage SP, Wright V. An objective clinical method to measure lateral spinal flexion. *Rheumatol Phys Med.* 1972;11:225-239.

18. O'Driscoll SL, Tomenson J. The cervical spine. *Clin Rheum Dis.* 1982;8:617-630.

19. Twomey L. The effects of age on the range of motion of the lumbar region. *Aust J Physiother.* 1979;25:257-263.

20. Youdas JW, Garrett TR, Suman VJ, Bogard CL, Hallman HO, Carey JR. Normal range of motion of the cervical spine: an initial goniometric study. *Phys Ther.* 1992; 72:770-780.

21. Buck CA, Dameron FB, Dow MJ, Skowlund HV. Study of normal range of motion in the neck utilizing a bubble goniometer. *Arch Phys Med Rehabil.* 1959;40:390-392.

22. Kuhlman KA. Cervical range of motion in the elderly. *Arch Phys Med Rehabil.* 1993;74:1071-1079.

23. Schoening HA, Hannan V. Factors related to cervical spine mobility. Part I. *Arch Phys Med Rehabil.* 1964;45:602-609.

24. Reid DC, Burnham RS, Saboe LA, Kushner SF. Lower extremity flexibility patterns in classical ballet dancers and their correlation to lateral hip and knee injuries. *Am J Sports Med.* 1987;15:347-352.

25. Bryant JT, Reid JG, Smith BL, Stevenson JM. Method for determining vertebral body positions in the sagittal plane using skin markers. *Spine.* 1989;14:258-265.

26. Pearcy MJ. Measurement of back and spinal mobility. *Clin Biomech.* 1986;1:44-51.

27. Pearcy MJ, Gill JM, Whittle MW, Johnson GR. Dynamic back movement measured using a three-dimensional television system. *J Biomech.* 1987;20:943-949.

28. Stokes IA, Bevins TM, Lunn RA. Back surface curvature and measurement of lumbar spinal motion. *Spine.* 1987;12:355-361.

29. Hellebrandt FA, Duvall EN, Moore ML. The measurement of joint motion: part III—reliability of goniometry. *Phys Ther Rev.* 1949;29:302-307.

30. Minor MA, Minor SD. *Patient Evaluation Methods for the Health Professional.* Reston, Va: Reston Publishing; 1985.

31. Salter N. Methods of measurement of muscle and joint function. *J Bone Joint Surg Br.* 1955;37B:474-491.

32. Waddell G. Personal communication. Sept 4, 1992.

33. Moore ML. The measurement of joint motion, part II: the techniques of goniometry. *Phys Ther Rev.* 1949; 29:256-264.

34. Gerhardt JJ, Rippstein JA. *Measuring and Recording of Joint Motion, Instrumentation and Techniques.* Toronto, Ontario: Hogrefe-Huber Publishers; 1990.

35. Fish DR, Wingate L. Sources of goniometric error at the elbow. *Phys Ther.* 1985;65:1666-1670.

36. Cole TM, Tobis JS. Measurement of musculoskeletal function: goniometry. In: Kottke FJ, Stillwell GK, Lehmann JF, eds. *Krusen's Handbook of Physical Medicine and Rehabilitation*. 3rd ed. Philadelphia, Pa: WB Saunders; 1982:19-33.

37. Rondinelli R, Murphy J, Esler A, Marciano T, Cholmakjian C. Estimation of normal lumbar flexion with surface inclinometry: a comparison of three methods. *Am J Phys Med Rehabil*. 1992;71:219-224.

38. Keeley J, Mayer TG, Cox R, Gatchel RJ, Smith J, Mooney V. Quantification of lumbar function. Part 5: reliability of range-of-motion measures in the sagittal plane and an in vivo torso rotation measurement technique. *Spine*. 1986;11:31-35.

39. Kottke FJ, Lehmann JF, eds. *Krusen's Handbook of Physical Medicine and Rehabilitation*. 4th ed. Philadelphia, Pa: WB Saunders; 1990.

40. Dvorak J, Panjabi MM, Chang DG, Theiler R, Grob D. Functional radiographic diagnosis of the lumbar spine: flexion-extension and lateral bending. *Spine*. 1991;16: 562-571.

41. Gill K, Krag MH, Johnson GB, Haugh LD, Pope MH. Repeatability of four clinical methods for assessment of lumbar spinal motion. *Spine*. 1988;13:50-53.

42. Mayer TG, Tencer AF, Kristoferson S, Mooney V. Use of noninvasive techniques for quantification of spinal range-of-motion in normal subjects and chronic low-back dysfunction patients. *Spine*. 1984;9:588-595.

43. Riddle DL, Rothstein JM, Lamb RL. Goniometric reliability in a clinical setting: shoulder measurements. *Phys Ther*. 1987;67:668-673.

44. Rothstein JM, Miller PJ, Roettger RF. Goniometric reliability in a clinical setting: elbow and knee measurements. *Phys Ther*. 1983;63:1611-1615.

45. Watkins MA, Riddle DL, Lamb RL, Personius WJ. Reliability of goniometric measurements and visual estimates of knee range of motion obtained in a clinical setting. *Phys Ther*. 1991;71:90-96.

46. American Academy of Orthopaedic Surgeons Committee for the Study of Joint Motion. *Joint Motion: Method of Measuring and Recording*. Chicago, Ill: American Academy of Orthopaedic Surgeons; 1965.

47. Russe OA, Gerhardt JJ, King PS. *An Atlas of Examination, Standard Measurements and Diagnosis in Orthopedics and Trauma*. Bern, Switzerland: Hans Huber Publishers; 1972.

48. Amis AA, Miller JH. The elbow. *Clin Rheum Dis*. 1982;8:571-593.

49. Bird HA, Stowe J. The wrist. *Clin Rheum Dis*. 1982;8:559-569.

50. Horger MM. The reliability of goniometric measurements of active and passive wrist motions. *Am J Occup Ther*. 1990;44:342-348.

51. Potney LG, Watkins MP. *Foundations of Clinical Research: Applications to Practice*. Norwalk, Conn: Appleton and Lange; 1993:505-528.

52. Shrout PE, Fleiss JL. Intraclass correlations: uses in assessing rater reliability. *Psychol Bull*. 1979;86:420-428.

53. Youdas JW, Bogard CL, Suman VJ. Reliability of goniometric measurements and visual estimates of ankle joint active range of motion obtained in a clinical setting. *Arch Phys Med Rehabil*. 1993;74:1113-1118.

54. Bohannon RW, Lieber C. Cybex II isokinetic dynamometer for passive load application and measurement: suggestion from the field. *Phys Ther*. 1986;66:1407.

55. Pandya S, Florence JM, King WM, Robinson JD, Oxman M, Province MA. Reliability of goniometric measurements in patients with Duchenne muscular dystrophy. *Phys Ther*. 1985;65:1339-1342.

56. Dvorak J, Panjabi MM, Grob D, Novotny JE, Antinnes JA. Clinical validation of functional flexion/extension radiographs of the cervical spine. *Spine*. 1993;18:120-127.

57. Flowers KR, Michlovitz SL. Assessment and management of loss of motion in orthopaedic dysfunction. In: *Postgraduate Advances in Physical Therapy*. Alexandria, Va: Physical Therapy Association; 1988:1-11.

58. Gerhardt JJ, Medeiros JM. *Objective Measurements and Documentation of Posture, Alignment and Joint Motion Textbook in Standardized Techniques, Numerical Documentation, New Instrumentation*. Portland, Ore: Isomed; 2002.

59. Lea RD, Gerhardt JJ. Current concepts in range-of-motion measurements. *J Bone Joint Surg Am*. 1995;77A:784-798.

60. Gowitzke BA, Milner M. *Understanding the Scientific Bases of Human Movement*. 2nd ed. Baltimore, Md: Williams and Wilkins; 1980.

How to Perform Joint Measurements in the Spine, Upper Extremities, and Lower Extremities

chapter 2

Measuring Joints in the Spine

ANATOMICAL AREA: CERVICAL SPINE

I. Preparation of Examinee: Refer to Part 1, page 4.

II. Anatomical Landmarks: Mark the T1 spinous process with a skin pencil or place a tape across it horizontally. Verify the position with an inclinometer. Locate the corner of the eye, upper ear attachment and the calvaria on the head.

III. Warm-up Exercises: Ask the examinee to extend and flex the neck, moving it forward and backward. Bend the neck laterally to the left and the right and rotate it to the left and right 3 times. Have him or her rotate the shoulders forward and backward 3 times, then move the shoulders up and down 3 times.

IV. SFTR Measurements Shown: A. Extension/flexion B. Left/right lateral bending C. Left/right rotation

Measuring in the sagittal plane (S)

Extension and flexion: cervical spine

A. S-Plane (extension -0- flexion)

Neutral -0- starting position: Examinee position

1. Establish the neutral -0- starting position
   a. The individual is seated in a chair with back support with one arm extended against a wall or tripod to prevent anterior or posterior movement of the trunk.
   b. The head is straight in both the sagittal and frontal planes.
   c. Stabilize the back against the backrest of the chair.
   d. Keep the individual's trunk steady while the individual moves through the motion of extension -0- and flexion.

Positioning and stabilization of the inclinometer

2. Position the inclinometer (Figure 2-1, Figure 2-2)
   a. Place the first inclinometer, set to the horizontal gravity -0- position, at the side of the face, from the corner of the eye to the upper attachment of the ear, along a parallel line where the temple of properly fit eyeglasses would sit.
   b. Tilt the head until the inclinometer shows 0.
   c. Place the second inclinometer over T1 or on the shoulder, and set it to 0 to monitor any movement of the trunk.
   d. Move the inclinometer to the calvaria without changing the position of the head or resetting the inclinometer.
   e. Spread the scalp between the thumb and fourth and fifth digits to prevent movement of the inclinometer with the scalp on the skull. The inclinometer should show 0 (starting position).

Extension: cervical spine

3. Measuring extension (Figure 2-3)
   a. Instruct the individual to extend the neck as far back as possible, recording both inclinometer angles.
   b. Ask the individual to return the head to the neutral -0- position.
   c. Repeat the extension measurement 2 more times.
   d. Subtract the T1 angle from the calvarium angle to obtain the cervical extension angle of each set.
   e. Ask the individual to return to the neutral -0- position.

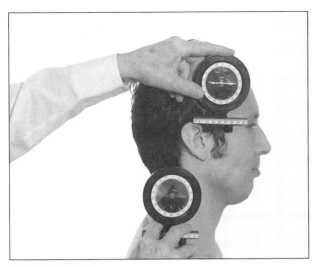

FIGURE 2-1

To establish the neutral -0- position of the cervical spine, tilt the examinee's head until the inclinometer, which is set to the horizontal gravity -0- position and placed on the eye-ear line, shows 0.

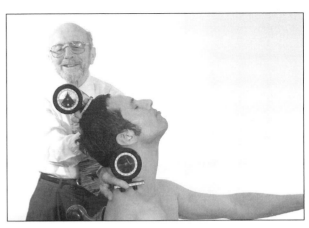

FIGURE 2-3

Measuring extension of the cervical spine.

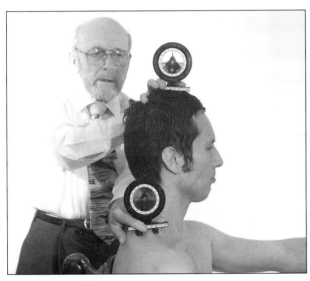

FIGURE 2-2

The inclinometer is transferred to the calvarium and stabilized at 0 degrees, without moving the examinee's head.

Flexion: cervical spine

4. Measuring flexion (Figure 2-4)
   a. Ask the individual to flex the neck maximally and record both angles. Make sure that the examinee keeps his/her chin close to the sternum to prevent anterior translation of the cervical spine.
   b. Ask the individual to return the head to the neutral -0- starting position.
   c. Repeat the flexion measurement 2 more times to assure validity.
   d. Subtract the T1 angle from the calvarium angle to obtain the true cervical flexion angle of each set.
   e. Ask the individual to return to the neutral -0- starting position.

Validation

5. Validation of rating
   a. The degrees of the 3 consecutive measurements should fall within 5° of one another or 10% of the mean to be valid.
   b. Use the greatest angles of extension and flexion of a valid set of three consecutive measurements for evaluation of impairment.

Recording

6. Recording
   Record the final motion of extension and flexion of the cervical spine:

   Cervical Spine: S: 60 -0- 50

   Note: If your individual state's rules require recording of the average reading, record the average reading rather than the highest reading.

Measuring in the frontal plane (F)

Left and right lateral bending: cervical spine

B. F-Plane (left lateral bending -0- right lateral bending)

Neutral -0- starting position:
Examinee position

1. Establish the neutral -0- starting position
   a. Examinee is sitting in a chair with a straight backrest with one arm abducted 90° against a tripod or wall to prevent lateral movement of the trunk.
   b. It is beneficial to place a portable mirror in front of the examinee so that both the examiner and the examinee can monitor their movements in the mirror to ensure there is no slippage of the inclinometer or concomitant rotation of the cervical spine.
   c. Both earlobes should be visible during left and right lateral bending, and the short extenders and the base of the inclinometer should always be parallel to the eye level line.
   d. Keep the individual's trunk steady while the individual moves through the motion of left and right lateral bending.
   e. The position of the head is the same as described in measuring extension and flexion in both the sagittal and frontal planes.

Positioning and stabilization of the inclinometer

2. Position the inclinometer (Figure 2-5)
   a. Place one inclinometer set to the horizontal gravity position aligned in the frontal plane over the T1 spinous process.
   b. Stabilize the second inclinometer over the calvarium. The head is in the neutral -0- position.
   c. Without moving the position of the body or head or resetting the inclinometers, place the inclinometers so that both show gravity 0.

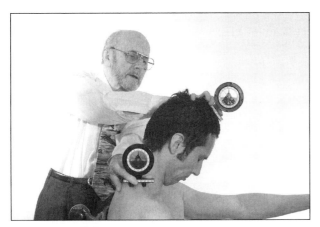

FIGURE 2-4

When measuring flexion of the cervical spine, have the examinee keep the chin close to the sternum.

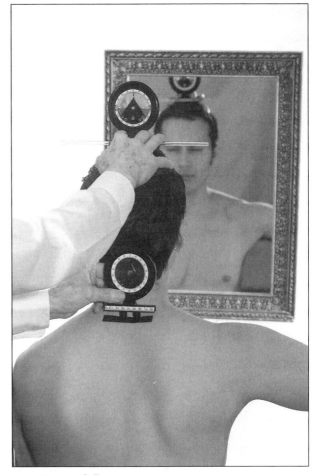

FIGURE 2-5

In neutral -0- starting position, both inclinometers, one on the calvarium and one over T1, read 0.

Left lateral bending: cervical spine

3. Measuring left lateral bending (Figure 2-6)
   a. Ask the individual to tilt the head maximally to the left and record both angles.
   b. Return the head to the neutral -0- starting position.
   c. Repeat measurement of left lateral bending 2 more times to assure reliability.
   d. Subtract the T1 angle from the calvarium angle to determine the degrees of left lateral bending.
   e. Return the head to the neutral -0- starting position.

Right lateral bending: cervical spine

4. Measuring right lateral bending
   a. Instruct the individual to tilt the head maximally to the right, recording both inclinometer angles.
   b. Ask the individual to return the head to the neutral -0- starting position.
   c. Tilt the head 2 more times to the right to assure validity.
   d. Subtract the T1 angle from the calvarium angle to determine cervical right lateral bending and record it.
   e. Return the head to the neutral -0- starting position

Validation

5. Validation of rating
   a. The three consecutive measurements should be within 5° of one another or 10% of the mean to be valid.
   b. Use the greatest angles of a valid set of three consecutive measurements of left and right lateral bending for evaluation of impairment.

Recording

6. Recording
   Record the range of motion of left and right lateral bending:

   Cervical Spine: F: 45 -0- 45

Measuring rotation (R)

Left and right rotation: cervical spine

C. Rotation (left rotation -0- right rotation)

Neutral -0- starting position
Examinee position

1. Establish the neutral -0- starting position
   a. The individual is in the supine position on the examining table. Ensure the individual's shoulders are stabilized on the table while rotating the head, to obtain only cervical rotation.

Positioning and stabilization of the inclinometer

2. Position the inclinometer (Figure 2-7)
   a. Only one inclinometer is needed. It is set to the gravity -0- position.
   b. Stand at the head of the table and place the inclinometer in the transverse plane on the forehead (vertical).
   c. Place the cupped free hand under the occiput to assure the individual is not rolling the head on the table but keeps the cervical spine straight (aligned with the spine). The individual's nose is pointing to the ceiling and the inclinometer reads 0.

Left rotation: cervical spine

3. Measuring left rotation (Figure 2-8)
   a. Ask the individual to rotate the head maximally to the left, and record the left cervical rotation angle.
   b. Return the head to the starting neutral -0- starting position.
   c. Repeat left rotation 2 more times to assure validity.
   d. Return to the neutral -0- starting position.

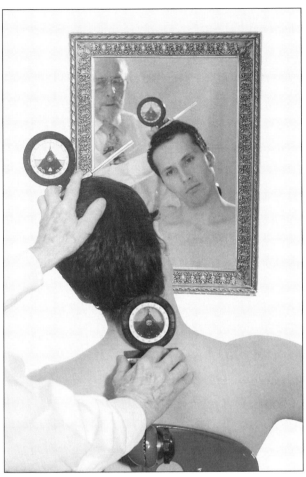

FIGURE 2-6

When measuring lateral bending of the cervical spine, avoid slippage of the inclinometer on the hair or skin.

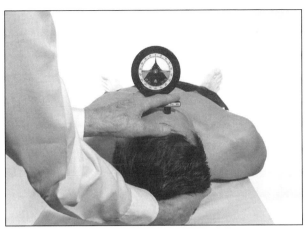

FIGURE 2-7

Neutral -0- starting position and stabilization of examinee for measuring right and left rotation of the cervical spine.

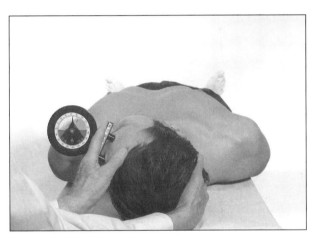

FIGURE 2-8

Measuring left rotation of the cervical spine of examinee in the supine position.

Right rotation: cervical spine

4. Measuring right rotation (Figure 2-9)
   a. Ask the individual to rotate the head maximally to the right, and record the cervical right rotation angle.
   b. Return to the neutral -0- starting position.
   c. Repeat the right rotation 2 more times to obtain a valid set of three consecutive measurements.
   d. Return to the neutral -0- starting position.

Validation

5. Validation of rating
   a. The 3 consecutive measurements should be within 5° of one another or 10% of the mean to be valid.
   b. Use the greatest angles of a valid set of three consecutive measurements of left and right cervical rotation for evaluation of impairment.

Recording

6. Recording
   Record the range of motion of left and right rotation:

   Cervical Spine: R: 80 -0- 80

V. Special Considerations

   A. Calibration of inclinometers to horizontal and vertical gravity positions
   See Part 1, page 10.

   B. Common Errors
   See Part 1, page 20.

   C. Conditions affecting ROM of the cervical spine
   See Part 1, page 19.

ANATOMICAL AREA: THORACIC SPINE

I. Preparation of Examinee: Refer to Part 1, page 4.

II. Anatomical Landmarks: Mark the T1 and T12 spinous processes with a pencil mark or place a tape across them horizontally. For information about how to find landmarks, refer to Part 1, page 4.

III. Warm-up Exercises: Refer to warm up exercises for spinal measurement: Part 1, page 5. Do the exercises described in numbers 1, 2, 3, 6, 7, 8, 9, 10, 11, 12, 18, and 19 or 20. Immediately before measurements are taken, extend and flex the spine 2 times, laterally bend the trunk left and right, and rotate the trunk to the left and right 2 times. Do the modified Thompson maneuver (20 seconds). Refer to Part 1, page 6, exercises 19 and 20.

IV. SFTR Measurements Shown: A. Extension/flexion B. Left/right rotation

Measuring in the sagittal plane (S)

Extension and flexion: thoracic spine

A. S-Plane (extension -0- flexion)

Neutral -0- starting position:
Examinee position

1. Establish the neutral -0- starting position
   a. Examinee is standing upright and relaxed. Two inclinometers are needed because the spine cannot be stabilized. The inclinometers will be placed at each end of the measured segment.

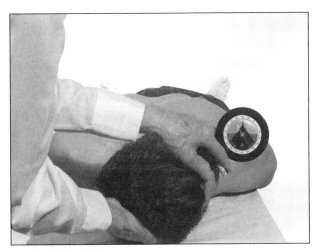

FIGURE 2-9

Measuring right rotation of the cervical spine of examinee in the supine position.

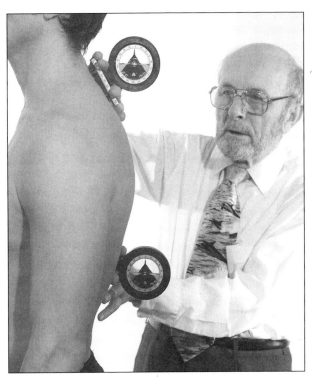

FIGURE 2-10

For neutral -0- starting position, or physiological kyphosis, the inclinometers are stabilized at the T1 and the T12 spinal processes.

Positioning and stabilization of
the inclinometer

2. Position the inclinometer (Figure 2-10)
   a. First place both inclinometers at the T12 level and set them to the
      0 position. (It is not a gravity -0- position.)
   b. Move one inclinometer to T1 and record the degree of the physiological
      kyphosis. Stabilize both inclinometers on the corresponding levels,
      cradling the spinous process T1 and T12 in the sagittal plane. For how to
      find landmarks, see Part 1, page 4.

Extension: thoracic spine
(minimal kyphosis)

3. Measuring extension (Figure 2-11)
   a. Ask the individual to extend the thoracic spine and read the values on
      both inclinometers.
   b. Return to the neutral -0- starting position.
   c. Repeat the extension 2 more times to obtain a valid reading.
   d. Subtract the T12 inclinometer reading from the T1 inclinometer reading
      to obtain the angle of extension or minimal kyphosis.
   e. Return to the neutral -0- starting position.

Flexion: thoracic spine

4. Measuring flexion (Figure 2-12)
   a. The inclinometer at T1 shows the degree of physiological kyphosis. The
      inclinometer at T12 should show 0 (or reposition the examinee until the
      T12 inclinometer shows 0 and the T1 the degree of physiological kypho-
      sis.) Ask the examinee to fully flex the thoracic spine. Flexing at the hips
      is permitted. Record both values.
   b. Return to the starting position.
   c. Repeat thoracic flexion 2 more times to obtain a valid reading.
   d. Read both values and subtract the T12 inclinometer reading from the T1
      reading to obtain the angle of thoracic flexion.

Validation

5. Validation of rating
   a. The 3 consecutive measurements should be within 5° of one another or
      10% of the mean to be valid.
   b. Use the greatest angles of extension and flexion of a valid set of three
      consecutive measurements for evaluation of impairment.

Recording

6. Recording
   Record the thoracic extension and flexion:

   Thoracic spine: S: 10 -0- 60

   (if the minimal kyphosis diminished to 10
   from the physiological value of 20)

Measuring rotation (R)

Left and right rotation: thoracic spine

B. Measuring rotation (left rotation -0- right rotation)

Neutral -0- starting position:
Examinee position

1. Establish the neutral -0- starting position
   a. Have the individual seated or standing, whichever is more comfortable,
      in a forward flexed position, with the thoracic spine in as horizontal a
      position as can be achieved.
   b. Use the previously placed horizontal skin marks over the T1 and T12
      spinous processes. The trunk should be in the neutral -0- starting position
      for rotation (shoulders horizontal).

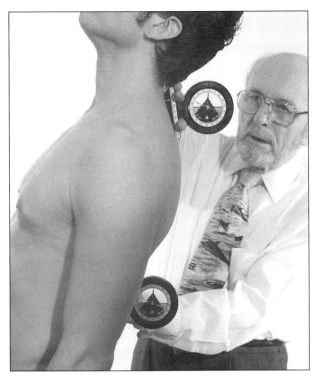

FIGURE 2-11

Measuring extension, or minimal kyphosis, of the thoracic spine. The inclinometers are stabilized at T1 and T12 in the sagittal plane.

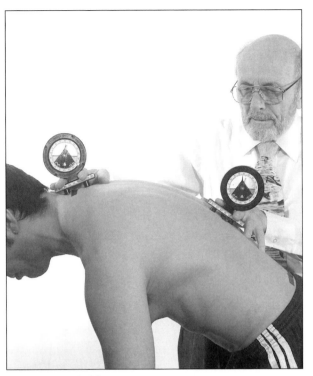

FIGURE 2-12

Measuring flexion of the thoracic spine. Keep the inclinometers stabilized at T1 and T12. Hip flexion is permitted.

Positioning and stabilization of
the inclinometer

2. Position the inclinometer (Figure 2-13)
   a. The inclinometers are set to the horizontal gravity -0- position. If they do
      not indicate gravity automatically, as is the case in most electronic incli-
      nometers, place the inclinometers against a flat, horizontal table or floor
      to calibrate them to horizontal gravity position. (See page 10 in Part 1.)
   b. Place the first inclinometer on the T1 mark in a vertical position and
      hold the second inclinometer over the T12 mark. Both inclinometers are
      placed across the spinal process in the frontal plane. Keep the inclinome-
      ters vertical.

Left rotation: thoracic spine

3. Measuring left rotation (Figure 2-14)
   a. Ask the individual to rotate the trunk maximally to the left
      (left shoulder up backwards) and record both angles.
   b. Return the trunk to the neutral -0- starting position.
   c. Repeat measurement of left rotation 2 more times to obtain a valid
      reading.
   d. Subtract the T12 angle from the T1 angle to obtain the thoracic left
      rotation angle.
   e. Return to the neutral -0- starting position.

Right rotation: thoracic spine

4. Measuring right rotation (Figure 2-15)
   a. Instruct the examinee to rotate the trunk maximally to the right, again
      recording both inclinometer angles.
   b. Return to the neutral -0- starting position.
   c. Repeat the measurement of right thoracic rotation 2 more times.
   d. Subtract the T12 angle from the T1 angle to obtain the thoracic right
      rotation angle.
   e. Return to the neutral -0- starting position.

Validation

5. Validation
   a. The degrees of the three consecutive measurements should be
      within 5° of one another or 10% of the mean to be valid.
   b. Use the greatest angles of left and right rotation for impairment
      evaluation.

Recording

6. Recording
   Record left and right rotation of the thoracic spine.

   Thoracic Spine: R: 30 -0- 30

V. Special Considerations

   A. Calibration of inclinometers
      See Part 1, page 10.

   B. Common Errors
      See Part 1, page 20.

   C. Conditions affecting ROM of the thoracic spine
      See Part 1, page 19.

   Note: If examinee cannot sufficiently bend forward, the inclinometers cannot
   be placed vertically and inaccurate or invalid measurements will be the conse-
   quence. In this case, an alternative technique of measuring rotation is offered.
   See *Guides*, Fifth Edition, page 415, and the described rotation of the
   thoraco-lumbar spine in supination that follows.

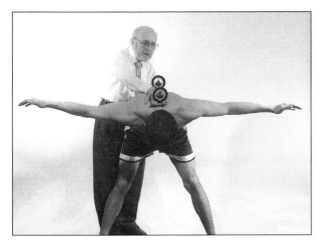

FIGURE 2-13

Measuring left and right rotation of the thoracic spine in the standing position. The examinee is bending forward; the inclinometers are in the horizontal gravity -0- position; and are stabilized at T1 and T12 in the frontal plane.

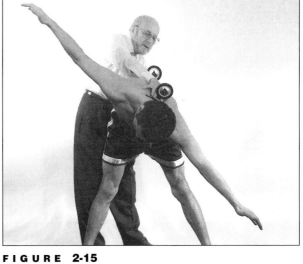

FIGURE 2-15

Measuring right rotation of the thoracic spine.

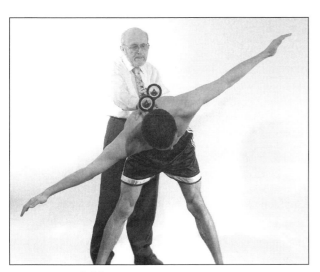

FIGURE 2-14

Measuring left rotation of the thoracic spine. Keep the bases of the inclinometers on the horizontal anatomical markers.

ALTERNATIVE TECHNIQUE FOR MEASURING THORACIC (THORACO-LUMBAR) ROTATION

Measuring rotation (R)

Left and right rotation: thoraco-lumbar spine

Measuring rotation (left rotation -0- right rotation)

Neutral -0- starting position: Examinee position	1. Establish the neutral -0- starting position a. The individual lies supine on the exam table. Stabilize the hips and pelvis.
Positioning and stabilization of the inclinometer	2. Position the inclinometer (Figure 2-16) a. Only one inclinometer, set to the horizontal gravity -0- position, is needed because the individual is in the supine position and stabilized on the examining table. If the examiner is able to hold the inclinometer with both hands, it can be stabilized on the manubrium, just below the sternal notch. Otherwise, the examiner stands behind the head of the examining table and stabilizes the inclinometer over the manubrium with both hands and the forearms close to both sides of the individual's head so there is no interference with the rotation. The trunk of the examinee should be in the neutral -0- starting position and the examinee should lift the elbow up during rotation.
Left rotation: thoraco-lumbar spine (supine)	3. Measuring left rotation a. Ask the individual to rotate the trunk maximally to the left and record the angle on the inclinometer, making certain an assistant holds the pelvis to the table without permitting rotation. Because the angle actually measures left thoraco-lumbar rotation, subtract 5°, the average lumbar rotation (1° per segment), to obtain the estimated thoracic rotation.
Right rotation: thoraco-lumbar spine (supine)	4. Measuring right rotation (Figure 2-17) a. Instruct the individual to rotate the trunk maximally to the right, again maintaining pelvic stabilization. Read the inclinometer angle and subtract 5° to obtain the right thoracic rotation angle.

Validation	5. Validation of rating
	  a. The degrees of the three consecutive measurements should be within 5° of one another or 10% of the mean to be valid.
	  b. Subtract 5° from the greatest angles of left and right thoraco-lumbar rotations (for the lumbar segment) then use the resulting values for evaluation of impairment of the thoracic spine, left and right rotation.

Recording	6. Recording Record left and right rotation of the thoraco-lumbar spine. **Thoraco-lumbar spine: R: 35 -0- 35** Now subtract 5° from each left and right rotation and record the adapted left and right rotation of the thoracic spine. **Thoracic spine: R: 30 -0- 30**

V. Special Considerations

A. Calibration of inclinometers. See Part 1, page 10.

B. Common errors. Inadequate stabilization of the pelvis and the inclinometer on the sternum. Keeping the shoulders down and not lifting the elbows off the table, thus obstructing rotation.

C. Conditions affecting ROM. See Part 1, page 19.

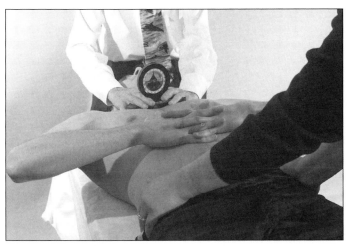

FIGURE 2-16

Neutral -0- starting position for measuring thoraco-lumbar rotation in the supine position. Only one inclinometer is needed. It is in the horizontal gravity -0- position and stabilized on the sternum.

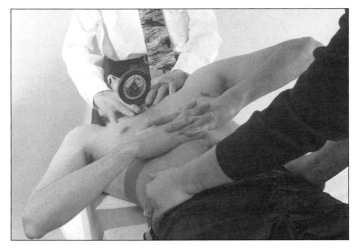

FIGURE 2-17

Right thoraco-lumbar rotation in the supine position. Note stabilization of the pelvis.

ANATOMICAL AREA: LUMBAR SPINE

I. Preparation of Examinee: Refer to Part 1, page 4.

II. Anatomical Landmarks: Use T1 – T12 from thoracic spine. Add S1, 2. Place mark or tape linking left and right PSIS (posterior, superior, iliac spines) just caudal to the dimples. (Corresponds with S2 level.) See Part 1, page 4.

III. Warm-up Exercises: See Part 1, page 5 for special warm-up exercises and Thompson maneuver. Do the exercises described by numbers 1, 2, 4, 5, 6, 7, 10, 11, 12, 18, 19, or 20.

IV. SFTR Measurements Shown: A. Extension/flexion B. Left/right lateral bending

Measuring in the sagittal plane (S)

Extension and flexion: lumbar spine

A. S-Plane (extension -0- flexion)

Neutral -0- starting position: Examinee position

1. Establish the neutral -0- starting position
   a. The individual should be standing with knees extended and weight balanced on both feet, ideally with hands on hips for support to permit greater motion. The spine should be in the neutral -0- starting position.

Positioning and stabilization of the inclinometer

2. Position the inclinometer (Figure 2-18)
   a. The first inclinometer is placed, in the sagittal plane, over the T12 spinous process. Center the second inclinometer over the S1 skin mark on the sacrum in the sagittal plane also. Set both inclinometers to 0. This is not a gravity -0- position.

Extension: lumbar spine

3. Measuring extension (Figure 2-19)
   a. Ask the individual to extend the lumbar spine maximally while holding the inclinometers firmly, and record both angles.
   b. Return the trunk to the neutral -0- starting position.
   c. Repeat the extension measurement 2 more times to obtain a valid reading.
   d. Subtract the sacral inclinometer angle from the T12 inclinometer angle to obtain the true lumbar extension angle.
   e. Return to the neutral -0- starting position.

Flexion: lumbar spine

4. Measuring flexion (Figure 2-20)
   a. Instruct the examinee to flex the trunk as far as possible, again recording both inclinometer angles.
   b. Ask the examinee to return the trunk to the neutral -0- starting position.
   c. Repeat flexion measurements 2 more times to obtain a valid reading.
   d. Return to the neutral -0- starting position.
   e. Subtract the sacral from the T12 inclinometer angle to obtain the true lumbar flexion angle.
   f. Return to the neutral -0- starting position.

Validation

5. Validation of rating
   a. The 3 consecutive measurements should be within 5° of one another or 10% of the mean to be valid. Only the true lumbar spine extension and flexion angles need to be consistently measured within 5° if the average is less than 50°, or within 10° if the average is greater than 50°.
   b. Use the greatest angles of extension and flexion from within the three consecutive measurements for impairment evaluation.

Recording

6. Recording
   Record lumbar spine extension -0- flexion:

Lumbar spine: S: 20 -0- 50

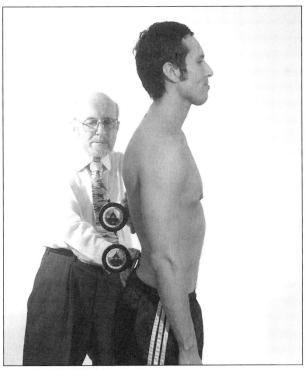

FIGURE 2-18

The inclinometers are stabilized at T12 and S1 and 2 in the sagittal plane and neutral -0- starting position. Set both inclinometers to 0.

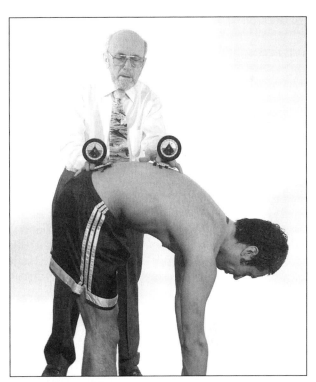

FIGURE 2-20

Flexion of the lumbar spine.

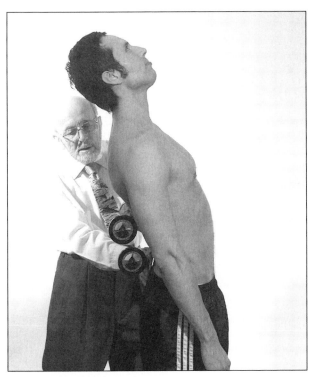

FIGURE 2-19

Extension of the lumbar spine.

Measuring in the frontal plane (F)

Left and right lateral bending: lumbar spine

B. F-Plane (left lateral bending -0- right lateral bending)

Neutral -0- starting position:
Examinee position

1. Establish the neutral -0- starting position
   a. With the examinee standing erect with knees extended, use the previously placed skin marks over T12 and S1 spinous processes. Verify with the inclinometer that the skin marks are truly horizontal (examinee is standing erect); do not rely solely on visual assessment. Both inclinometers are set to the horizontal gravity -0- position. The trunk should be in the upright neutral -0- starting position.

Positioning and stabilization of
the inclinometer

2. Position the inclinometer (Figure 2-21)
   a. Place the first inclinometer aligned in the frontal (coronal) plane over the T12 spinous process and hold the second over the sacrum. The inclinometers show horizontal gravity 0.

Left lateral bending: lumbar spine

3. Measuring left lateral bending (Figure 2-22)
   a. Instruct the examinee to bend the trunk laterally to the left and record both angles.
   b. Ask the examinee to return to the neutral -0- starting position.
   c. Repeat the procedure 2 more times to obtain a valid reading.
   d. Subtract the sacral inclinometer angle from the T12 inclinometer angle to determine the left lateral bending angle.
   e. Return to the neutral -0- starting position.

Right lateral bending: lumbar spine

4. Measuring right lateral bending (Figure 2-23)
   a. Instruct the examinee to bend the trunk to the right as far as possible. Record both inclinometer angles.
   b. Ask the examinee to return to the neutral -0- starting position.
   c. Repeat the procedure 2 more times to obtain a valid reading.
   d. Return to the neutral -0- starting position.
   e. Subtract the sacral angle from the T12 inclinometer angle to obtain the right lumbar lateral bending angle.
   f. Return to the neutral -0- starting position.

Validation

5. Validation of rating
   a. The 3 consecutive measurements should be within 5° of one another or 10% of the mean to be valid.
   b. Use the greatest angles of left and right lateral bending of the lumbar spine from a valid set for evaluation of impairment.

Recording

6. Recording
   Record the left and right lateral bending of the lumbar spine.

   Lumbar spine: F: 30 -0- 30

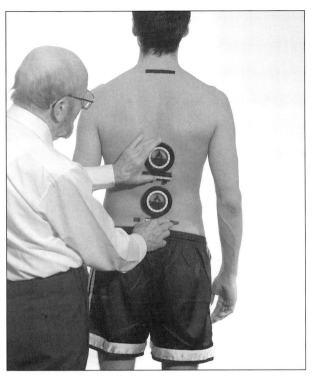

FIGURE 2-21

The inclinometers are stabilized at T12 and S1 and 2 in the frontal plane and are in the horizontal gravity -0- position. Do not set the inclinometers to 0, but adjust the position of the examinee so the inclinometers read 0.

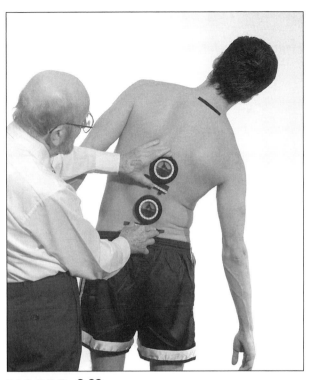

FIGURE 2-23

Right lateral bending.

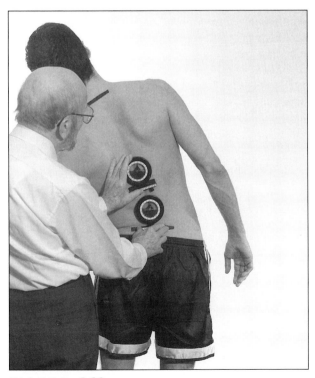

FIGURE 2-22

Left lateral bending. Keep the bases of the inclinometers perpendicular to the spine (on the horizontal anatomical markers).

Straight Leg Raising (SLR)

Validity check for extension/flexion of the lumbar spine

C. SLR—Validity check

Neutral -0- starting position: Examinee position

1. Establish the neutral -0- starting position
   a. The straight leg raising is done to assess validity of the lumbar spine extension and flexion movements. The examinee is in the supine position on the examining table with knees straight.

Positioning and stabilization of the inclinometer

2. Position the inclinometer (Figure 2-24)
   a. Place one inclinometer on the distal tibial crest or align the extender with the lateral axis of the leg and set it to 0.

SLR

3. Measuring SLR (Figure 2-25)
   a. Lift the straight leg passively to the tightest position and read the angle of the straight leg raising.
   b. Repeat 2 more times for reliability.
   c. Return to the neutral -0- starting position.
   d. Repeat straight leg raising on opposite leg. Read the angle and repeat 2 more times for reliability.
   e. Return to the neutral -0- starting position.

Validation

4. Validation of rating
   a. The degrees of the 3 consecutive measurements on each side should be within 5° of one another or 10% of the mean to be valid.
   b. Compare the straight-leg-raising angle of the tightest side to the sum of the sacral extension and flexion (sacral or hip motion) angles. If the straight-leg-raising angle exceeds the sum of sacral flexion and extension angles by more than 15°, the lumbosacral extension/flexion test of the lumbar spine is invalid. If the test is invalid, the examiner should either repeat the extension/flexion test or disallow impairment for lumbosacral spine extension and flexion.

   Note: Tightest SLR - (sacral flexion + sacral extension) is less than or equal to 15° for validity (assumes sacral flexion and extension are less than normal). This accessory validity test is useful only when sacral flexion plus extension is less than the average for normal individuals (ie, 65° for women and 55° for men). See *Guides,* Fifth Edition, page 406.

Recording

5. Recording
   Record the left and right tightest straight-leg-raising angle:

   Right SLR: S: 0-70
   Left SLR: S: 0-60

   Note: The numbers represent the position in the tightest angle, not flexion at the hip.

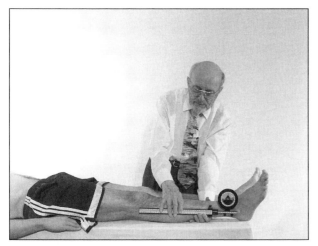

FIGURE 2-24

Neutral -0- starting position for measuring straight leg raising. The extender is aligned along the lateral axis of the leg.

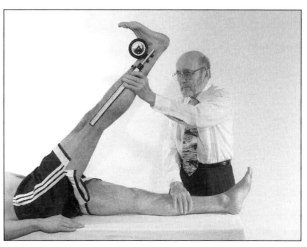

FIGURE 2-25

The straight leg is raised to the tightest position for hip flexion. Hold the opposite extremity down to prevent hip flexion.

chapter 3

Measuring Joints in the Upper Extremities

To measure the motion of the large joints in the extremities, it is best to attach an extender (either rigid or telescopic) to the base of the inclinometer rather than using the two-arm conventional goniometer. It improves accuracy because the inclinometer allows accurate and measured determination of the starting position related to gravity, while the conventional goniometer relies on visual assessment and maintenance of the stationary arm in the visually assessed position. The extender converts the inclinometer into a single-arm goniometer (Figure 3-1).

ANATOMICAL AREA: SHOULDER

I. Preparation of Examinee: Refer to Part 1, page 4.

II. Anatomical Landmarks: Locate the acromion, olecranon, lateral epicondyle of humerus, styloid of radius, distal ulna, the long axes of the arm (posterior, lateral, anterior) and the forearm.

III. Warm-up Exercises: Have the examinee go through the motion of full extension and flexion, abduction and adduction, and external and internal rotation slowly four times. Also see Part 1, pages 5, 6, exercise numbers 1, 2, 3, 6, 7, 9, and 18.

IV. SFTR Measurements Shown: A. Extension/flexion B. Abduction/adduction C. External/internal rotation

Measuring in the sagittal plane (S)

Extension and flexion: shoulder

A. S-Plane (extension -0- flexion)

Neutral -0- starting position:
Examinee position

1. Establish the neutral -0- starting position
   a. Place the examinee in neutral -0- starting position, standing or sitting in a chair with the backrest against the back, one arm braced against a wall or tripod in front of the body to prevent anterior/posterior movement of the trunk. For measuring extension of the shoulder, the arm is at the side of the body, with the forearm in mid-position between supination and pronation and the palm facing the thigh.

Positioning and stabilization of the inclinometer and extender

2. Positioning the inclinometer and extender (Figure 3-2)
   a. Set the inclinometer to the vertical gravity -0- position with the extender aligned with the long axis of the arm.

Extension of the shoulder

3. Measuring extension (Figure 3-3)
   a. Ask the examinee to extend the arm back as far as possible, keeping the trunk straight. Read the degrees of extension.
   b. Ask the examinee to return to the neutral -0- starting position with the arm at the side.
   c. Repeat the procedure 2 more times to obtain a valid reading.
   d. Ask the examinee to return to the neutral -0- starting position.

Flexion of the shoulder

4. Measuring flexion (Figure 3-4)
   a. Ask the individual to flex the shoulder maximally. Keep the alignment of the extender along the long axis of the arm. Read and record the angle of flexion.
   b. Ask the examinee to return the arm to the neutral -0- starting position.
   c. Repeat the procedure 2 more times to obtain a valid reading.
   d. Ask the examinee to return to the neutral -0- starting position.

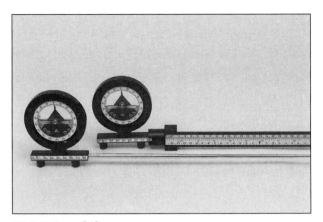

FIGURE 3-1

A bar with swivel and telescopic extender with inclinometers.

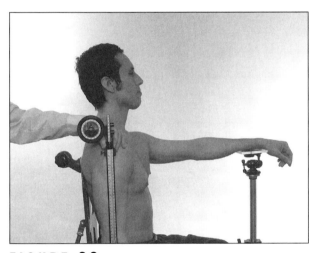

FIGURE 3-2

The shoulder is in the neutral -0- starting position in the sagittal plane.

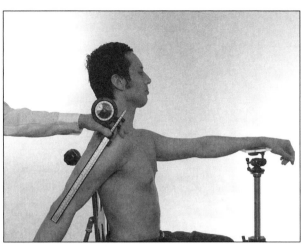

FIGURE 3-3

Measuring extension of the shoulder in the sagittal plane.

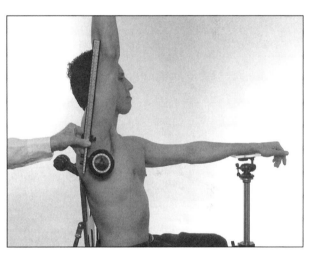

FIGURE 3-4

Measuring flexion of the shoulder in the sagittal plane.

Validation

5. Validation of rating
   a. The 3 consecutive measurements should be within 5° of one another or 10% of the mean to be valid.
   b. Use the greatest angle of extension and flexion for rating.

Recording

6. Recording
   Record the extension and flexion of the shoulder. Indicate the side: right or left.

   Right shoulder: S: 50 -0- 180

   Alternative method
   a. The extension and flexion of the shoulder can also be measured in the supine position. The examinee is in supine position on the examining table, with the shoulder and arm extended beyond the margin of the table. This method adds stability to the body.
   b. The motion of extension is toward the floor and the motion of flexion toward the ceiling and the cranium.
   c. Record the repetitions and validity check in the same way whether the examinee is in the standing or sitting position.

Measuring in the frontal plane (F)

Shoulder abduction/adduction

B. F-Plane: (abduction -0- adduction in 30° flexion)

Neutral -0- starting position
Examinee position

1. Establish the neutral -0- starting position
   a. Ask the examinee to stand or sit with the trunk upright. The arm is in anatomical neutral -0- position at the side of the body, palm facing anteriorly. Ask the examinee to abduct the opposite arm to 90° and brace it against a wall or tripod to prevent left or right lateral motion of the trunk (in the frontal plane).

Positioning the inclinometer
and extender

2. Position the inclinometer and extender (Figure 3-5)
   a. Set the inclinometer, attached to an extender, to vertical gravity -0- position. Stand behind the examinee and align the extender with the long axis of the arm. This is the neutral -0- starting position.

Abduction of the shoulder

3. Measuring abduction (Figure 3-6)
   a. Ask the examinee to abduct the arm maximally. Keep the extender aligned along the long axis of the arm even if the arm rotates during this motion (Codman's paradox). Read the degrees of abduction.
   b. Ask the examinee to return to the neutral -0- starting position.
   c. Repeat the procedure 2 more times to obtain a valid reading.
   d. Ask the examinee to return to the neutral -0- starting position.

Adduction of the shoulder

4. Measuring adduction (See page 53.)
   Adduction of the shoulder is blocked by the body. It can be measured only if the arm is in a certain degree of flexion, which varies greatly from individual to individual because of anatomy, body build, obesity, pregnancy, etc. We propose to set a standard of 30° of flexion in which to measure adduction.

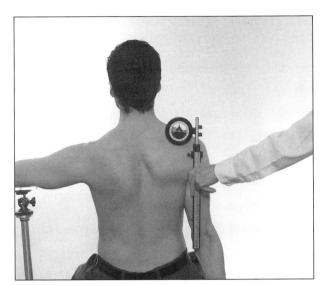

FIGURE 3-5

The shoulder is in the neutral -0- starting position in the frontal plane.

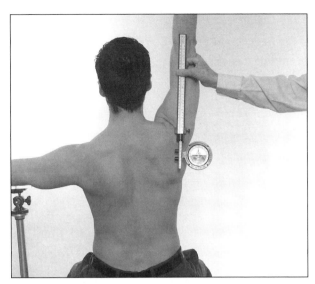

FIGURE 3-6

Abduction of the shoulder in the frontal plane.

a. The following are instructions for measuring adduction in a standing position. (To measure adduction in a sitting position as shown, the examinee must flex the elbow to 90° to allow the arm to move in front of the body.) To set flexion of the shoulder at 30°, stand at the side of the examinee and ask the examinee to rotate the forearm into mid-position, between supination and pronation (the thumb facing anteriorly). Align the extender with the long axis of the arm, and ask the examinee to flex the arm to 30°.

b. Move in front of the examinee and align the extender with the long axis of the arm in the frontal plane. However, place the inclinometer end of the extender somewhat away from the arm, to maintain the inclinometer in the vertical position. Place the arm so the inclinometer shows gravity 0. Ask the examinee to adduct the arm in front of the body and read the degree of adduction in 30° of flexion. (Figures 3-7, 3-8, 3-9). Ask the examinee to return to the neutral -0- starting position in the frontal plane.

c. Repeat the procedure 2 more times to obtain a valid reading.

d. Ask the examinee to return to the neutral -0- starting position.

Validation

5. Validation of rating
    a. The 3 consecutive measurements should be within 5° of one another or 10% of the mean to be valid.
    b. Use the greatest angle of abduction and adduction for rating purposes.

Recording

6. Recording
    Record right shoulder abduction and adduction (in 30° of flexion) as F. Next, record the degrees of flexion in parentheses after the degrees of adduction with the initial S (sagittal) for flexion.

    Right shoulder: F: 160 -0- 30 (S30)

Measuring shoulder rotation (R)

External rotation/internal rotation: shoulder

C. Measuring rotation (external rotation -0- internal rotation)

Neutral -0- starting position
Examinee position

1. Establish neutral -0- starting position
    a. Standard rotation is done in 90° of shoulder abduction with the elbow flexed 90° and the forearm serving as an indicator of rotation. The examinee is sitting or supine with the arm stabilized on the table and the elbow and forearm are placed beyond the margin of the table with the forearm pronated. When sitting, the arm is supported on a tripod or narrow table.

Positioning and stabilization
of the inclinometer and extender

2. Position the inclinometer and extender (Figure 3-10)
    a. Neutral -0- starting position is when the forearm is vertical in the supine position and horizontal in sitting position.
    b. Align the extender along the long axis of the forearm, with the attached inclinometer set to horizontal gravity -0- position if the examinee is sitting or vertical gravity -0- position if the examinee is in the supine position.

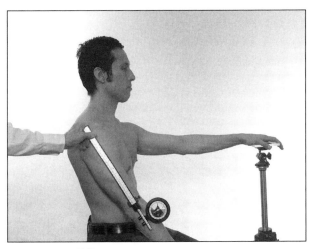

FIGURE 3-7

Preparation of the shoulder for measuring adduction, setting arm in flexion of 30° in the sagittal plane.

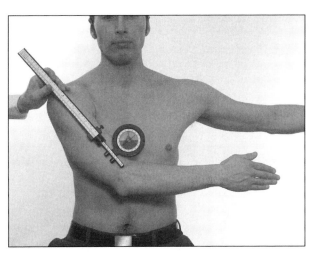

FIGURE 3-9

Adduction of the shoulder in 30° of flexion.

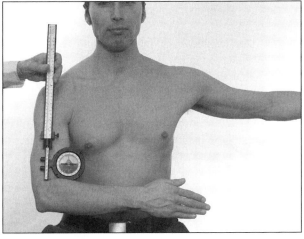

FIGURE 3-8

Preparation of the shoulder for measuring adduction in flexion of 30°. This is the neutral -0- starting position in the frontal plane.

External rotation of the shoulder

3. Measuring external rotation (Figure 3-11)
    a. Ask the examinee to externally rotate the shoulder (the forearm moves cranially in the supine position and toward the ceiling in the sitting position). Read and record the degrees of external rotation.
    b. Ask the examinee to return to the neutral -0- starting position.
    c. Repeat the procedure 2 more times to obtain a valid reading.
    d. Ask the examinee to return to the neutral -0- starting position.

Internal rotation of the shoulder

4. Measuring internal rotation
    a. Ask the examinee to internally rotate the shoulder (forearm moves toward the table in supine position and toward the floor in the sitting position). Read and record the degrees of internal rotation.
    b. Ask the examinee to return to the neutral -0- starting position.
    c. Repeat the procedure 2 more times to obtain a valid reading.
    d. Ask the examinee to return to the neutral -0- starting position.

Validation

5. Validation of rating
    a. The 3 consecutive measurements should be within 5° of one another or 10% of the mean to be valid.
    b. Use the greatest (least impairing) angle of external and internal rotation for rating.

Recording

6. Recording
    a. Record the degrees of external and internal rotation with the shoulder abducted 90°. Place (F90) after the initial R (rotation), which indicates rotation in 90° shoulder abduction.

Right shoulder: R (F90): 90 -0- 90

Note: Because the shoulder rotation can be measured in other positions than in 90° of shoulder abduction, it is necessary to record the shoulder abduction when recording external and internal rotation. Record the abduction of the shoulder in parenthesis after the initial *R* for rotation, with the initial *F* for abduction.

If rotation is measured with the arm at the side of the body it has to be measured in the supine position so the forearm is vertical to allow vertical placement of the inclinometer.

Right shoulder: R(F0): 30 -0- 45
F0=0 abduction of the shoulder

Note: In the standing or sitting position with the arm abducted 90°, the forearm is horizontal in the starting position. The upper arm must be properly supported in 90° abduction on a tripod or high narrow table so the elbow, flexed to 90°, can be placed beyond the edge of the arm support to allow movement of the forearm. Align the extender along the long axis of the forearm, with the attached inclinometer set to the horizontal gravity -0- position.

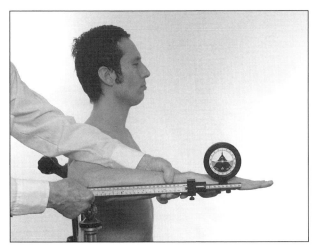

FIGURE 3-10

The shoulder is in neutral -0- starting position for measuring rotation (sitting with arm stabilized).

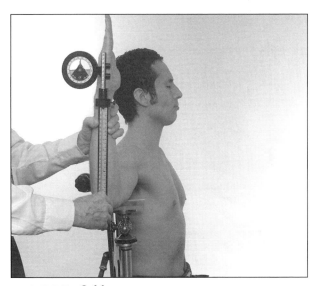

FIGURE 3-11

Measuring external rotation of the shoulder.

ANATOMICAL AREA: ELBOW

I. Preparation of Examinee: Refer to Part 1, page 4.

II. Anatomical Landmarks: Locate the greater tuberosity of the humerus, the lateral epicondyle of the humerus, the styloid process of the radius, and the long axes of the arm and the forearm.

III. Warm-up Exercises: Extend and flex the elbows slowly 4 times, supinate and pronate the elbows slowly 4 times. See Part 1, pages 5, 6, exercise numbers 1, 2, 3, 8, 9, and 17.

IV. SFTR Measurements Shown: Extension/flexion

Measuring in the sagittal plane (S)

Extension and flexion: elbow

A. S-Plane: (extension -0- flexion)

Neutral -0- starting position
Examinee position

1. Establish the neutral -0- starting position
   a. The examinee is in the supine or sitting position with the arm of the measured side stabilized on the examining table or a treatment table. The elbow and the supinated forearm are beyond the margin of the table to allow free motion of the elbow.

Positioning and stabilization
of the inclinometer and extender

2. Position the inclinometer and extender (Figure 3-12)
   a. Set the inclinometer to the horizontal gravity -0- position. Align the extender along the long axis of the forearm and position the forearm so the inclinometer reads 0.

Hyper-extension of the elbow

3. Measuring hyper-extension
   a. If the examinee is able to hyper-extend the elbow, read and record the degrees of hyper-extension on the left side of neutral 0.
   b. Ask the examinee to return to the neutral -0- starting position. If there is no hyper-extension, record 0 on the left side of neutral 0.
   c. Repeat the procedure 2 more times to obtain a valid reading.
   d. Ask the examinee to return to the neutral -0- starting position.

Flexion of the elbow

4. Measuring flexion (Figure 3-13)
   a. Ask the examinee to maximally flex the elbow and maintain the alignment of the extender along the long axis of the forearm. Read and record the degrees of flexion on the right side of neutral 0.
   b Ask the examinee to return to the neutral -0- starting position.
   c. Repeat the procedure 2 more times to obtain a valid reading.
   d. Ask the examinee to return to the neutral -0- starting position.

Validation

5. Validation of rating
   a. The 3 consecutive measurements should be within 5° of one another or 10% of the mean to be valid.
   b. Use the greatest angle of hyper-extension and flexion for rating.

Recording

6. Recording
   a. Record extension (hyper-extension and flexion). Indicate side: left or right.

   Right elbow: S: 0 -0- 135 (extension is 0)

   Right elbow: S: 10 -0- 135 (with hyper-extension of 10 degrees)

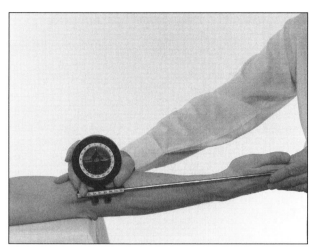

FIGURE 3-12

The elbow is in the neutral -0- starting position. Note the use of a telescopic extender.

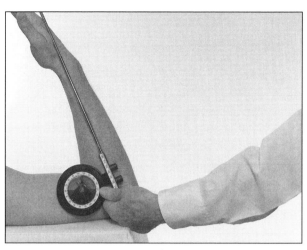

FIGURE 3-13

Measuring flexion of the elbow. Note the use of a telescopic extender.

ANATOMICAL AREA: FOREARM

I. Preparation of Examinee: Refer to Part 1, page 4.

II. Anatomical Landmarks: Locate the elbow, wrist, hand, thumb, palm, and the distal palmar crease of the wrist, (rascetta). Also, see Part 1, Page 4, Figure 1-2.

III. Warm-up Exercises: Extend and flex the elbows slowly 4 times, then supinate and pronate the forearms slowly 4 times. Also see Part 1, pages 5, 6, exercise numbers: 1, 2, 3, and 17.

IV. SFTR Measurements Shown: Supination/pronation

Measuring rotation (R)

Supination and pronation: forearm

A. Measuring rotation: (supination -0- pronation)

Neutral -0- starting position
Examinee position

1. Establish the neutral -0- starting position
   a. Have the examinee sit in a chair with the arm of the measured side stabilized against the side of the body and the forearm in mid-position between supination and pronation (thumb up, palm facing the midline of the body) and elbow flexed 90°. Brace the opposite arm in 90° abduction against a wall, chair, or tripod to prevent lateral movement of the trunk.

Positioning and stabilization
of the inclinometer

2. Position the inclinometer (Figure 3-14)
   a. Set the inclinometer to vertical gravity -0- position. If the examinee is able to hold the inclinometer in the measured-side hand, ask the examinee to hold the base of the inclinometer in the measured hand, in vertical gravity position so the inclinometer shows 0 when the measured forearm is in the neutral -0- starting position.
   b. If the examinee is unable to hold the inclinometer, see the alternative technique below.

Supination of the forearm

3. Measuring supination (Figure 3-15)
   a. Ask the examinee to supinate the forearm maximally (rotate the palm toward the ceiling). Read and record the degrees of supination.
   b. Ask the examinee to return to the neutral -0- starting position.
   c. Repeat the procedure 2 more times to obtain a valid reading.
   d. Ask the examinee to return to the neutral -0- starting position.

Pronation of the forearm

4. Measuring pronation (Figure 3-16)
   a. Ask the examinee to pronate the forearm maximally (rotate the palm toward the floor). Read and record the degrees of pronation.
   b. Ask the examinee to return to the neutral -0- starting position.
   c. Repeat the procedure 2 more times to obtain a valid reading.
   d. Ask the examinee to return to the neutral -0- starting position.

Validation

5. Validation
   a. The 3 consecutive measurements should be within 5° of one another or 10% of the mean to be valid.
   b. Use the greatest (least impairing) angle of supination and pronation for rating.

Recording

6. Recording
   Record supination and pronation of the forearm. Indicate the side: right or left.

Right forearm: R: 90 -0- 90

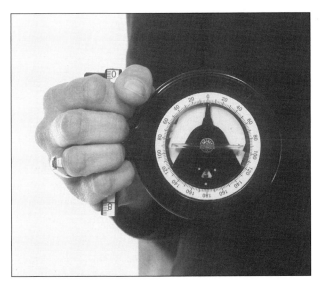

FIGURE 3-14

Neutral -0- starting position of the forearm for measuring supination and pronation. Examinee is holding the base of the inclinometer.

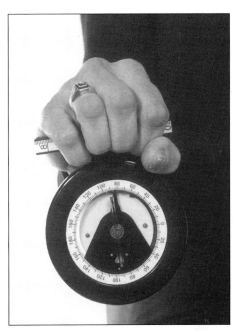

FIGURE 3-16

Measuring pronation of the forearm (palm is facing down).

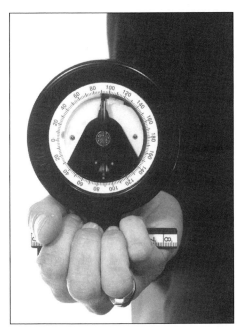

FIGURE 3-15

Measuring supination of the forearm (palm is facing up).

Alternative measuring technique

Supination and pronation: forearm

	B. Alternative measuring technique Measuring rotation: (supination -0- pronation)
Neutral -0- starting position Examinee position	1. Establish the neutral -0- starting position a. Have the examinee sit in a chair with the arm of the measured side stabilized against the side of the body and the forearm in mid-position between supination and pronation (the thumb up, the palm facing the midline of the body) and the elbow flexed 90°. Brace the opposite arm in 90° abduction against a wall, chair, or tripod to prevent lateral movement of the trunk.
Positioning and stabilization of the inclinometer	2. Position the inclinometer (Figure 3-17) a. If the examinee is not able to hold the inclinometer in the hand on the measured side, the examiner applies the inclinometer over the distal skin fold of the wrist (rascetta), which corresponds with the proximal row of the carpal bones.

Supination of the forearm	3. Measuring supination (Figure 3-18)
	   a. The examiner asks the examinee to actively supinate the forearm and then records the angle of supination.
	   b. The individual returns the forearm to the neutral -0- starting position.
	   c. Repeat the supination 2 more times to assure validity.
	   d. Ask the individual to return the forearm to the neutral -0- starting position.

Pronation of the forearm	4. Measuring pronation
	   a. Ask the examinee to maximally pronate the forearm and record the angle of pronation.
	   b. Ask the individual to return to the neutral -0- starting position.
	   c. Pronate the forearm 2 more times to assure validity.
	   d. Ask the individual to return to the neutral -0- starting position.

Validation	5. Validation of rating
	   a. The degrees of 3 consecutive measurements should fall within 5° of one another or 10% of the mean to be valid.
	   b. Use the greatest angle of supination and pronation of a valid set of 3 consecutive measurements for rating.

Recording	6. Recording a. Record active motion of supination-pronation. Identify the side: right or left. **Right forearm: R: 90 -0- 90** Note: When using this technique, the examiner has to be careful not to influence the active motion of supination and pronation of the forearm of the examinee.

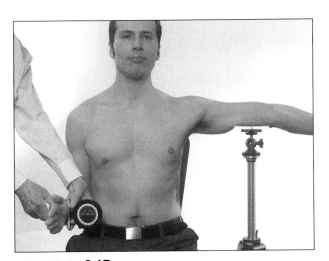

FIGURE 3-17

The forearm is in the neutral -0- starting position. The palm is facing the body.

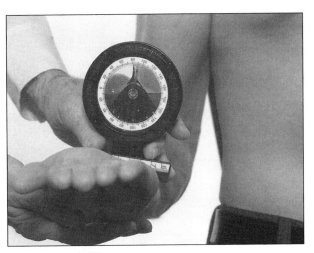

FIGURE 3-18

Measuring supination of the forearm. The palm faces up.

ANATOMICAL AREA: WRIST

I. Preparation of Examinee: Refer to Part 1, page 4.

II. Anatomical Landmarks: Locate the wrist, forearm, third metacarpal-dorsal and volar side, digit III, the long axes of the forearm and the third metacarpal, the thenar, and the hypothenar. See Part 1, page 4, Figure 1-1.

III. Warm-up Exercises: Extend and flex the elbows slowly 4 times; extend and flex the wrist slowly 4 times. Radial deviation (up) and ulnar deviation (down) in midposition between supination and pronation. Also see Part 1, page 6, exercise number 17.

IV. SFTR Measurements Shown: A. Extension (dorsiflexion)/flexion (volar flexion) B. Radial/ulnar deviation

Measuring in the sagittal plane (S)

Extension and flexion: wrist

A. S-Plane: (extension -0- flexion)

Neutral -0- starting position
Examinee position

1. Establish the neutral -0- starting position
   a. Ask the examinee to sit in a chair next to a table, with the pronated forearm and the hand (palm down) on the table.

Positioning and stabilization
of the inclinometer

2. Position the inclinometer (Figure 3-19)
   a. Set the inclinometer to the horizontal gravity -0- position, and place it on the long axis of the third metacarpal bone on the dorsal side.
   b. Set the inclinometer to 0.
   c. Ask the examinee to move the forearm forward so that the hand and wrist extend beyond the margin of the table, to allow free motion of the wrist.
   d. Maintain the wrist angle at -0- as indicated by the inclinometer. This is the neutral -0- starting position.

Extension (dorsiflexion) of the wrist

3. Measuring extension (dorsiflexion) (Figure 3-20)
   a. Ask the examinee to extend (dorsiflex) the wrist maximally (the motion is toward the ceiling). Maintain the stabilization of the inclinometer on the third metacarpal during the motion. Read and record degrees of extension.
   b. Ask the examinee to return to the neutral -0- starting position.
   c. Repeat the procedure 2 more times to obtain a valid reading.
   d. Ask the examinee to return to the neutral -0- starting position.

Flexion (palmar flexion) of the wrist

4. Measuring flexion
   a. Ask the examinee to flex the wrist maximally (the motion is toward the floor). Maintain the stabilization of the inclinometer on the third metacarpal during the motion. Read and record the degrees of flexion.
   b. Ask the examinee to return to the neutral -0- starting position.
   c. Repeat the procedure 2 more times to obtain a valid reading.
   d. Ask the examinee to return to the neutral -0- starting position.

Validation

5. Validation of rating
   a. The 3 consecutive measurements should be within 5° of one another or 10% of the mean to be valid.
   b. Use the greatest angle of extension and flexion of a valid set of 3 consecutive measurements for rating.

Recording

6. Recording
   Record extension and flexion of the wrist.

Right wrist: S: 60 -0- 50

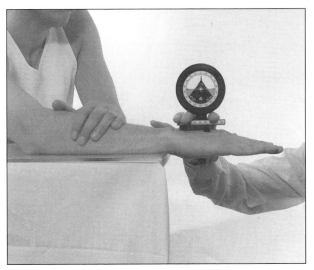

FIGURE 3-19

The wrist is in neutral -0- starting position in the sagittal plane.

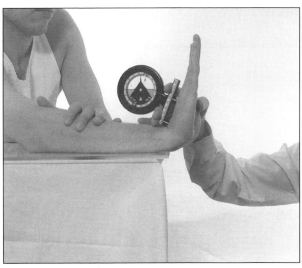

FIGURE 3-20

Measuring extension (dorsiflexion) of the wrist.

Measuring in the frontal plane (F)

Radial and ulnar deviation: wrist

B. F-Plane: (radial deviation -0- ulnar deviation)

Neutral -0- starting position
Examinee position

1. Establish the neutral -0- starting position
   a. Ask the examinee to sit on a chair beside a table with the forearm stabilized on the table. The forearm is in mid-position between supination and pronation (thumb up), with the hand resting on the table on the hypothenar and the little finger.

Positioning and stabilization
of the inclinometer

2. Position the inclinometer (Figure 3-21)
   a. Place the base of the inclinometer on the long axis of the third metacarpal, MC III (palmar side), which is aligned with the long axis of the forearm and the third digit, and set it to 0. Ask the examinee to move the forearm forward beyond the margin of the table to assure free motion of the wrist in the frontal plane. Align the wrist so the inclinometer still indicates 0. This is the neutral -0- starting position. Ask the examinee to stabilize the measured forearm on the table in the frontal plane by holding it down with the free hand.

Radial deviation of the wrist

3. Measuring radial deviation (Figure 3-22)
   a. Ask the examinee to move the hand toward the ceiling to place the wrist in maximal radial deviation. Read and record the degrees of radial deviation.
   b. Ask the examinee to return to the neutral -0- starting position.
   c. Repeat the procedure 2 more times to obtain a valid reading.
   d. Ask the examinee to return to the neutral -0- starting position.

Ulnar deviation of the wrist

4. Measuring ulnar deviation
   a. Ask the examinee to move the hand toward the floor to place the wrist in maximal ulnar deviation. Read and record the degrees of ulnar deviation.
   b. Ask the examinee to return to the neutral -0- starting position.
   c. Repeat the procedure 2 more times to obtain a valid reading.
   d. Ask the examinee to return to the neutral -0- starting position.

Validation

5. Validation of rating
   a. The 3 consecutive measurements should be within 5° of one another or 10% of the mean to be valid.
   b. Use the greatest (least impairing) angles of radial and ulnar deviation for ratings.

Recording

6. Recording
   Record radial and ulnar deviation of the wrist. Indicate the side: left or right.

   Right wrist: F: 20 -0- 30

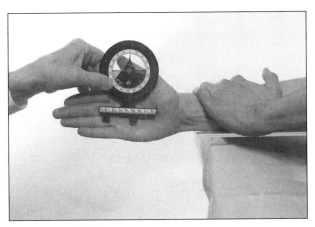

FIGURE 3-21

The wrist is in neutral -0- starting position in the frontal plane for measuring wrist deviation.

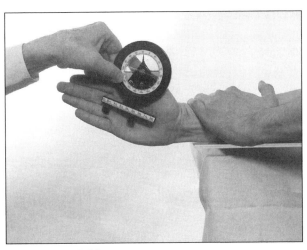

FIGURE 3-22

Measuring radial deviation of the wrist in the frontal plane.

ANATOMICAL AREA: HAND (THUMB AND DIGITS)

Hand Stabilization Devices

To accurately measure the joints of the hand, improvised or commercially available hand stabilization devices are needed. The average tables, examining tables, or desks are inadequate because the thickness of the cover plate precludes measuring flexion of the joints of the digits greater than 90°. Stabilization is also substandard.

A simple plastic or glass plate with rounded edges not thicker than ¼ inch can be purchased inexpensively, placed on top of a table or desk, and serve as an acceptable stabilization device. Another option would be a ¼ inch thick cutting board of proper size to accommodate placement of the forearm with hand. The plate or cutting board must be flat on the table, sturdy, and protrude about 3 inches beyond the table to allow proper stabilization of the proximal component and free movement of the distal component of the measured joint (Figure 3-23).

A hand-stabilization device is also available commercially that allows proper stabilization of the proximal component of the joints of the wrist and digits for measurement of extension and flexion. It also offers the advantage of making it easier to measure radial and ulnar deviation of the wrist and abduction and adduction of the digits without using inclinometers (Figure 3-24).

Planes of Motion of the Thumb

The thumb is positioned uniquely at a 45° angle to the basic planes and the carpometacarpal joint I (CMC I) moves in two directions (saddle joint). Therefore, the movements in this joint have to be recorded in two vectors: one in the frontal plane (VF) or radial abduction and the other in the sagittal plane (VS) or palmar abduction. Adduction and opposition are best measured functionally in centimeters.

ANATOMICAL AREA: CARPOMETACARPAL I JOINT OF THE THUMB (CMC I)

I.   Preparation of Examinee: Refer to Part 1, page 4.

II. Anatomical Landmarks: Locate the joints of the thumb and digits, the interphalangeal crease of the thumb, the distal palmar crease, and the long axes of the metacarpals and digits. See Part 1, page 4, Figure 1-2.

III. Warm-up Exercises: See Part 1, page 6, exercise number 17.

IV. SFTR Measurements Shown: A. VF radial (long) abduction and adduction in centimeters B. VS palmar (short) abduction, circumduction, and opposition in centimeters.

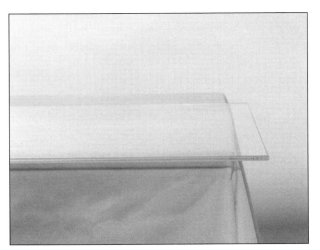

FIGURE 3-23

One-quarter-inch thick stabilization plate on a table.

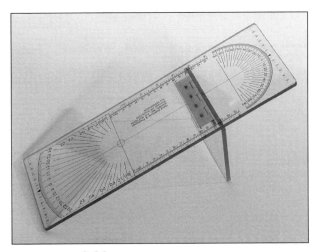

FIGURE 3-24

A hand stabilization device (HSD) on a table.

Measuring in the frontal plane (VF)

Radial abduction and adduction: thumb

A. VF-Plane: (radial abduction -0- adduction)

Neutral -0- starting position
Examinee position

1. Establish the neutral -0- starting position
   a. Radial abduction is measured in relation to the second metacarpal. The forearm and the hand are placed on the ulnar side with the forearm in mid-position between supination and pronation.

Positioning and stabilization
of the inclinometer

2. Position the inclinometer (Figure 3-25)
   a. The base of the inclinometer is aligned parallel to the long axis of the second metacarpal bone and set to 0. This is the neutral -0- starting position.

Radial abduction (VF) of the thumb
(CMC I)

3. Measuring radial abduction (Figure 3-26)
   a. Ask the examinee to maximally abduct the thumb (move the thumb toward the ceiling). Align the inclinometer with the long axis of the first metacarpal bone and read and record the radial abduction angle of the thumb.
   b. Return the thumb toward the second metacarpal.
   c. Repeat the motion of radial abduction 2 more times to obtain a valid reading.
   d. Ask the individual to return to the neutral -0- starting position.

Adduction of the thumb (CMC I)

4. Measuring adduction (Figure 3-27)
   a. Place the forearm and the hand on the stabilization plate on the ulnar side. Bring the thumb as close as possible to the second digit and adduct it maximally across the palm toward the little finger, keeping the interphalangeal joint of the thumb straight.
   b. Measure the smallest distance between the flexor interphalangeal crease of the thumb and the midline axis of the fifth metacarpal bone as it crosses the distal palmar crease in centimeters.
   c. Return the thumb to the neutral -0- starting position.
   d. Repeat the procedure 2 more times to obtain a valid reading of the thumb adduction.
   e. Return to the neutral -0- starting position.

Validation

5. Validation of rating
   a. The degrees of the 3 consecutive measurements should be within 5° of one another or 10% of the mean to be valid.
   b. Use the greatest angle of abduction and smallest distance of adduction (least impairing values) for rating.

Recording

6. Recording
   Record the abduction and adduction of the thumb in the CMC I joint.

   Right thumb
   Right CMC I VF: 50 -0- 2 cm

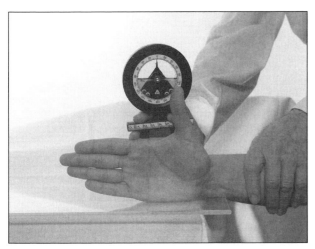

FIGURE 3-25

Neutral -0- starting position for measuring radial abduction of the carpometacarpal joint of the thumb (CMC I) in the frontal plane. It is recorded as VF. The inclinometer is at 0 on the second metacarpal.

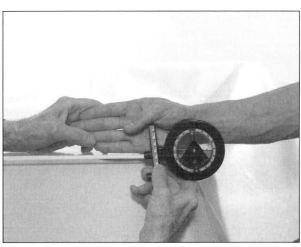

FIGURE 3-27

Measuring thumb adduction in centimeters; the IPP is extended and the MCP I is flexed.

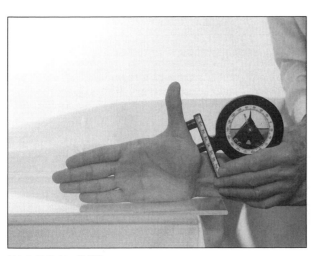

FIGURE 3-26

Measuring radial abduction of the thumb at the carpometacarpal I joint (CMC I) in the frontal plane. It is recorded as VF. The inclinometer is on the first metacarpal (MC I).

Opposition of the thumb

Through circumduction into maximal palmar abduction (VS)

B. Measuring opposition of the thumb

To measure opposition of the thumb, first have the examinee circumduct the thumb until it reaches maximal palmar abduction (VS) and beyond until it opposes the third digit.

Neutral -0- starting position
Examinee position

1. Establish the neutral -0- starting position
   a. Place the forearm and the hand in supination on the stabilization plate (palm up).

Positioning and stabilization
of the inclinometer

2. Position the inclinometer (Figure 3-28)
   a. Place the inclinometer on the second metacarpal and set it to 0.

Palmar abduction (VS) of the thumb

3. Measuring palmar abduction (Figure 3-29)
   a. Ask the examinee to circumduct the thumb in front of the second digit and abduct it maximally in the sagittal plane. Align the inclinometer with the long axis of the first metacarpal bone, and read and record the palmar abduction angle (VS).
   b. Return to the neutral -0- starting position.
   c. Repeat VS measurement 2 more times to obtain a valid reading of palmar abduction.
   d. Return to the neutral -0- starting position.

Opposition of the thumb in centimeters

4. Measuring opposition of the thumb (CMC I joint) (Figure 3-30)
   a. Ask the examinee to further circumduct the thumb from maximal palmar abduction until it opposes the third digit. Keep the first metacarpophalangeal joint and the interphalangeal joint of the thumb extended. Measure the largest distance between the flexor interdigital crease of the thumb and the distal palmar crease at the point of intersection with the long axis of the third metacarpal in centimeters.
   b. Return to the neutral -0- starting position.
   c. Repeat the procedure 2 more times to obtain a valid reading of the opposition of the thumb.
   d. Return to the neutral -0- starting position.

Validation

5. Validation of rating
   a. The 3 consecutive measurements should be within 5° of one another or 10% to be valid.
   b. Use the greatest angle of the palmar abduction and greatest distance of opposition (between the interphalangeal crease of the thumb and the cross point on the long axis of the hand and distal palmar crease).

Recording

6. Recording
   Record the opposition of the thumb as the greatest VS abduction angle in degrees and greatest linear distance of active opposition in centimeters.

Opposition of the thumb

R: VS 50 -0- 8 cm

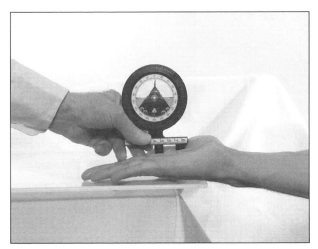

FIGURE 3-28

Neutral -0- starting position for measuring palmar abduction with the inclinometer zeroed out on the second metacarpal (MC II).

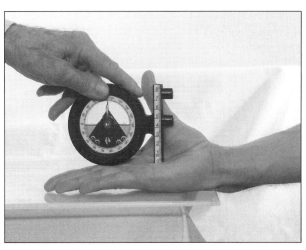

FIGURE 3-30

Measuring circumduction/opposition of the thumb in centimeters.

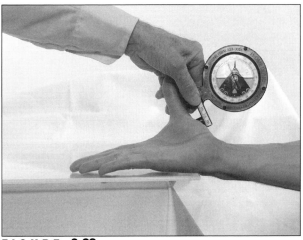

FIGURE 3-29

Measuring palmar abduction with the inclinometer on the first metacarpal (MC I). It is recorded as VS.

ANATOMICAL AREA: METACARPOPHALANGEAL JOINT OF THE THUMB (MCP I)

I. Preparation of Examinee: Refer to Part 1, page 4.

II. Anatomical Landmarks: Locate the metacarpophalangeal joint I (MCP I), carpometacarpal joint I (CMC I), the interphalangeal joint of the thumb, the metacarpals I and II, the phalanges of digits I, II, and V, the long axis of the hand and digits I, II, III, and V, the interphalangeal flexor crease of the thumb, the distal palmar crease, and the thenar. See Part 1, page 4, Figure 1-2.

III. Warm-up Exercises: See Part 1, page 6, exercise number 17.

IV. SFTR Measurements Shown: A. Extension/flexion

Measuring in the sagittal plane (S)

A. S-Plane: (extension -0- flexion)

Neutral -0- starting position:
Examinee position

1. Establish the neutral -0- starting position
   a. Place the thumb of the examinee close to the margin of the stabilization plate so that the entire thumb and the first metacarpal are stabilized on the plate and the hand is beyond the margin of the plate.

Positioning and stabilization
of the inclinometer

2. Position the inclinometer (Figure 3-31)
   a. Place the inclinometer on the proximal phalanx of the thumb.
   b. Set it to 0°.
   c. Ask the examinee to move the hand forward so that the MCP I joint is beyond the margin of the stabilization plate and allows free motion.
   d. Position the proximal phalanx until the inclinometer shows 0°.
   e. The examinee stabilizes the first metacarpal on the plate by pressing it down. This is the neutral -0- starting position for measuring extension and flexion in the MCP I joint of the thumb.

Extension of the thumb in the MCP I
joint

3. Measuring extension
   a. Ask the examinee to maximally extend the thumb in the MCP I joint (moving the proximal phalanx up). Read and record the extension angle.
   b. Return to the neutral -0- starting position.
   c. Repeat the procedure 2 more times to obtain a valid reading of extension.
   d. Return to the neutral -0- starting position.

Flexion of the thumb in the MCP II
joint

4. Measuring flexion (Figure 3-32)
   a. Ask the examinee to flex the thumb maximally in the MCP joint (the motion is down). Read and record the angle of flexion in the MCP I joint.
   b. Return to the neutral -0- starting position.
   c. Repeat the procedure 2 more times to obtain a valid reading of flexion.
   d. Return to the neutral -0- starting position.

Validation

5. Validation of rating
   a. The degrees of the 3 consecutive measurements should be within 5° of one another or 10% of the mean to be valid.
   b. Use the greatest angle of extension and flexion of a valid set of 3 measurements for rating.

Recording

6. Recording
   Record extension (hyper-extension) and flexion of the thumb in the MCP I joint.

Right MCP I: S: 0 -0- 60

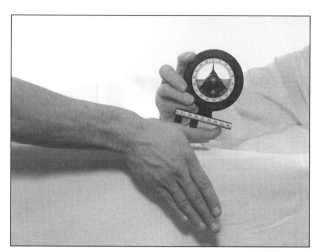

FIGURE 3-31

Neutral -0- starting position with the inclinometer on 0 on the proximal phalanx of the thumb in the sagittal plane.

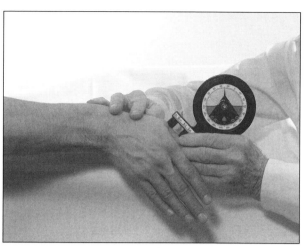

FIGURE 3-32

Measuring flexion of the metacarpophalangeal joint of the first digit (MCP I).

ANATOMICAL AREA: INTERPHALANGEAL JOINT OF THE THUMB (IPP)

I. Preparation of Examinee: Refer to Part 1, page 4.

II. Anatomical Landmarks: Locate the proximal and distal phalanges of the thumb, the interphalangeal joint (IPP), the metacarpophalangeal joint of the first digit (MCP I), the long axis of the thumb, and the thenar. Also see Part 1, page 4, Figure 1-2.

III. Warm-up Exercises: Move all the joints of the thumb through a full range of motion 4 times. See Part 1, page 6, exercise number 17.

IV. SFTR Measurements Shown: A. Extension/flexion

Measuring in the sagittal plane (S)

A. S-Plane (extension -0- flexion)

Neutral -0- starting position Examinee position	1. Establish the neutral -0- starting position a. Place the hand of the examinee the same way as in measuring extension and flexion of the MCP I joint. Stabilize the inclinometer on the distal phalanx of the thumb.

Positioning and stabilization of the inclinometer	2. Position the inclinometer
	   a. Set the inclinometer to 0°.
	   b. Ask the examinee to move the hand forward so that only the interphalangeal joint of the thumb (IPP) is beyond the margin of the table and can move freely through extension and flexion.
	   c. Position the end phalanx so that the inclinometer shows 0. This is the neutral -0- starting position for measuring the IPP joint.
	   d. Have the examinee stabilize the proximal phalanx of the thumb by pressing it down on the stabilization plate.
	   e. Return to the neutral -0- starting position.

Extension of the thumb in the IPP joint	3. Measuring extension
	   a. Ask the examinee to maximally extend the distal phalanx. Read and record the extension in the IPP joint.
	   b. Return to the neutral -0- starting position.
	   c. Repeat the extension measurement 2 more times to obtain valid readings.
	   d. Return to the neutral -0- starting position.

Flexion of the thumb in the IPP joint	4. Measuring flexion (Figure 3-33)
	   a. Ask the examinee to maximally flex the thumb in the IPP joint and read and record the flexion angle.
	   b. Return to the neutral -0- starting position.
	   c. Repeat the flexion measurement 2 more times to obtain valid readings.
	   d. Return to the neutral -0- starting position.

Validation	5. Validation of rating
	   a. The degrees of the 3 consecutive measurements should be within 5° of one another or 10% of the mean to be valid.
	   b. Use the greatest angle of extension and flexion of a valid set of 3 consecutive measurements for rating.

Recording	6. Recording Record extension (hyper-extension) and flexion in the IPP joint of the thumb.

Right thumb: IPP: S 30 -0- 80

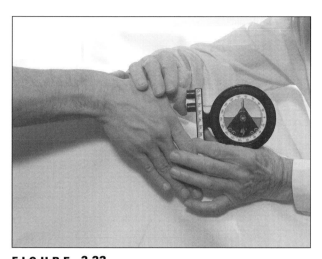

FIGURE 3-33

Measuring flexion of the interphalangeal joint of the thumb (IPP).

ANATOMICAL AREA: METACARPOPHALANGEAL JOINT OF THE SECOND DIGIT (MCP II)

I. Preparation of Examinee: See Part 1, page 4.

II. Anatomical Landmarks: Locate the the metacarpal I (MC I), the phalanges of the index finger, the metacarpophalangeal joint of the second digit (MCP II), the proximal interphalangeal joint of the second digit (PIP II), the distal interphalangeal joint of the second digit (DIP II), the long axis of the metacarpal II, and digit II. See Part 1, page 4.

III. Warm-up Exercises: Move all the joints of the index finger through extension and flexion slowly 4 times. Also, see Part 1, page 6, exercise number 17.

IV. SFTR Measurements Shown: A. Extension/flexion B. Abduction/adduction (optional)

Measuring in the sagittal plane (S)

Extension and flexion of the MCP II

A. S-Plane: (extension -0- flexion)

Neutral -0- Starting position Examinee position	1. Establish the neutral -0- starting position a. Ask the examinee to sit on a chair beside a table with the forearm, hand and fingers prone on a stabilization device. Move the legs of the inclinometer to one side, and close enough to fit on the proximal phalanx of the second digit.

Positioning and stabilization of the inclinometer	2. Position the inclinometer (Figure 3-34)
	   a. Stabilize the inclinometer on the proximal phalanx of the second digit, and set the inclinometer to 0.
	   b. Ask the examinee to move the forearm and the hand forward until the metacarpophalangeal joint of the second digit (MCP II) is beyond the margin of the stabilization device to allow free motion of the joint.
	   c. Align the digit until the inclinometer shows 0. This is the neutral -0- starting position.
	   d. Ask the examinee to stabilize the hand (metacarpal bone II) by holding it down with the free hand.

Extension (dorsiflexion) of the index finger (digit II) in the MCP II joint	3. Measuring extension (dorsiflexion) (Figure 3-35)
	   a. Ask the examinee to extend the MCP II maximally (motion is toward the ceiling). Read and record the degree of extension.
	   b. Ask the examinee to return to the neutral -0- starting position.
	   c. Repeat the procedure 2 more times to obtain a valid reading.
	   d. Ask the examinee to return to the neutral -0- starting position.

Flexion of the index finger (digit II) in the MCP II joint	4. Measuring flexion (Figure 3-36)
	   a. Ask the examinee to flex the MCP II maximally (the motion is toward the floor). Read and record the degree of flexion.
	   b. Ask the examinee to return to the neutral -0- starting position.
	   c. Repeat the procedure 2 more times to obtain a valid reading.
	   d. Ask the examinee to return to the neutral -0- starting position.

Validation	5. Validation of rating
	   a. The 3 consecutive measurements should be within 5° of one another or 10% of the mean to be valid.
	   b. Use the greatest (least impairing) degree of extension and flexion for rating.

Recording	6. Recording Record extension and flexion in the MCP joint of the left second digit (index finger):

Left MCP II: S: 20 -0- 90

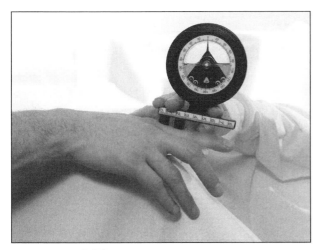

FIGURE 3-34

Neutral -0- starting position of the metacarpophalangeal joint of the second digit (MCP II).

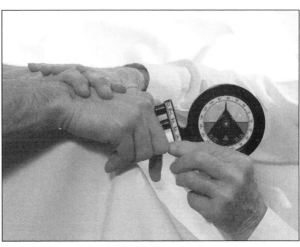

FIGURE 3-36

Measuring flexion of the metacarpophalangeal joint of the second digit (MCP II).

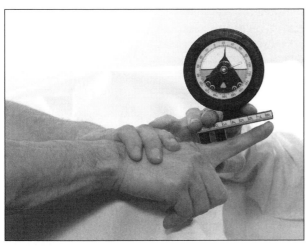

FIGURE 3-35

Measuring extension of the metacarpophalangeal joint of the second digit (MCP II).

ANATOMICAL AREA: PROXIMAL INTERPHALANGEAL JOINT OF THE SECOND DIGIT (PIP II)

I. Preparation of Examinee: See Part 1, page 4.

II. Anatomical Landmarks: Locate the metacarpal II, the proximal phalanx of digit II, the metacarpophalangeal joint of the second digit (MCP II), the proximal interphalangeal joint (PIP II), the long axis of the second metacarpal, and the index finger.

III. Warm-up Exercises: Extend and flex all the joints of the index finger 4 times slowly. See Part 1, page 6, exercise number 17.

IV. SFTR Measurements Shown: A. Extension/flexion

Measuring in the sagittal plane (S)

Extension and flexion in the PIP II

A. S-Plane: (extension -0- flexion)

Neutral -0- starting position Examinee position	1. Establish the neutral -0- starting position a. Ask the examinee to sit on a chair beside a table with the forearm, hand, and fingers prone on a stabilization device. Move the legs of the inclinometer to one side, and close enough to fit on the proximal phalanx of the second digit.

Positioning and stabilization
of the inclinometer
	2. Position the inclinometer
	   a. Stabilize the inclinometer on the middle phalanx of the second digit, and set the inclinometer to 0.
	   b. Ask the examinee to move the forearm and hand forward until the proximal interphalangeal joint of the second digit (PIP II) is beyond the margin of the stabilization device to allow free motion of the joint.
	   c. Align the digit until the inclinometer shows 0. This is the neutral -0- starting position.
	   d. Ask the examinee to stabilize the hand and the proximal phalanx of the second digit by holding them down with the free hand.

Extension of the index finger (digit II)
in the PIP joint
	3. Measuring extension (PIP II)
	   a. Ask the examinee to extend the PIP II maximally (motion is toward the ceiling). Read and record the degree of extension. Normally the degree of extension is 0. If there is extension, it is called hyper-extension.
	   b. Ask the examinee to return to the neutral -0- starting position.
	   c. Repeat the procedure 2 more times to obtain a valid reading.
	   d. Ask the examinee to return to the neutral -0- starting position.

Flexion of the index finger (digit II)
in the PIP joint
	4. Measuring flexion (Figure 3-37)
	   a. Ask the examinee to flex the PIP joint II maximally (the motion is toward the floor). Read and record the degree of flexion.
	   b. Ask the examinee to return to the neutral -0- starting position.
	   c. Repeat the procedure 2 more times to obtain a valid reading.
	   d. Ask the examinee to return to the neutral -0- starting position.

Validation	5. Validation of rating
	   a. The 3 consecutive measurements should be within 5° of one another or 10% of the mean to be valid.
	   b. Use the greatest angles of extension (hyper-extension) and flexion for rating.

Recording	6. Recording Record extension and flexion in the PIP joint of the left second digit (index finger):

Left PIP II: S: 0 -0- 100

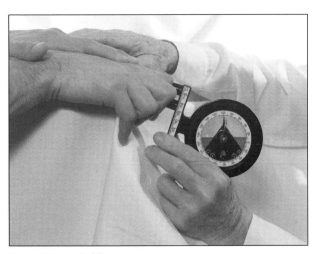

FIGURE 3-37

Measuring flexion of the proximal interphalangeal joint of the second digit (PIP II).

ANATOMICAL AREA: DISTAL INTERPHALANGEAL JOINT OF THE SECOND DIGIT (DIP II)

Measuring in the sagittal plane (S)

Extension and flexion in the DIP II

A. S-Plane: (extension -0- flexion)

Neutral -0- starting position
Examinee position

1. Establish the neutral -0- starting position
   a. Ask the examinee to sit on a chair beside a table with the forearm, hand, and fingers prone on a stabilization device. Move the legs of the inclinometer to one side, and close enough to fit on the distal phalanx of the second digit.

Positioning and stabilization
of the inclinometer

2. Position the inclinometer
   a. Stabilize the inclinometer on the distal phalanx of the second digit.
   b. Set the inclinometer to 0.
   c. Ask the examinee to move the forearm and the hand forward until the distal interphalangeal joint (DIP II) is beyond the margin of the stabilization device to allow free motion of the joint. Stabilize middle phalanx.
   d. Align the digit until the inclinometer shows 0. This is the neutral -0-starting position.

Extension of the index finger (digit II)
in the DIP joint

3. Measuring extension
   a. Ask the examinee to extend the DIP II maximally (motion is toward the ceiling). Read and record the degree of extension. Normally the degree of extension is 0. If there is extension, it is called hyper-extension.
   b. Ask the examinee to return to the neutral -0- starting position.
   c. Repeat the procedure 2 more times to obtain a valid reading.
   d. Ask the examinee to return to the neutral -0- starting position.

Flexion of the index finger (digit II)
in the DIP joint

4. Measuring flexion (Figure 3-38)
   a. Ask the examinee to flex the DIP II joint maximally (the motion is toward the floor). Read and record the degree of flexion.
   b. Ask the examinee to return to the neutral -0- starting position.
   c. Repeat the procedure 2 more times to obtain a valid reading.
   d. Ask the examinee to return to the neutral -0- starting position.

Validation

5. Validation of rating
   a. The 3 consecutive measurements should be within 5° of one another or 10% of the mean to be valid.
   b. Use the greatest angle of extension and flexion of the DIP II joint for rating.

Recording

6. Recording
   Record extension and flexion of the DIP joint of the left second digit (index finger):

   Left DIP II: S: 0 -0- 100

   Measurements of digits III, IV, and V are taken in the same fashion as the presented measurements of digit II.

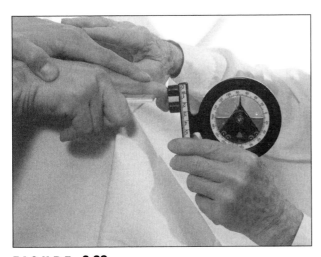

F I G U R E   3-38

Measuring flexion of the distal interphalangeal joint of the
second digit (DIP II).

Measuring Joints in the Lower Extremities

ANATOMICAL AREA: HIP

I. Preparation of Examinee: Refer to Part 1, page 4.

II. Anatomical Landmarks: Identify the trochanter, the lateral condyle of the femur, the patella, the anterior superior iliac spine (ASIS), the long axes of the thigh in the sagittal and frontal planes, the tibial crest, and the long axes of the leg and foot (the middle of the heel through the second toe).

III. Warm-up Exercises: Stand beside a chair and hold onto the chair with one hand, flex the hip and the knee, return to the neutral -0- starting position, and repeat 2 times. Next, extend the hip back, keeping the body straight, then return to the neutral -0- starting position and repeat 2 times. Rotate the foot from the hip, in and out, keeping the leg straight 2 times. Switch sides and repeat. Also, refer to Part 1, pages 5, 6, exercise numbers 1, 4, 5, 10, 11, 12, 13, 14, 19, and 20.

IV. SFTR Measurements Shown: A. Extension/flexion B. Abduction/adduction C. External/internal rotation

Measuring in the sagittal plane (S)

Extension and flexion: hip

A. S-Plane: (extension -0- flexion)

Neutral -0- starting position
Examinee position

1. Establish the neutral -0- starting position
   a. For measuring hip extension, the trunk and the pelvis are in the prone position on the examining table. One hip is flexed beyond the table to 90° and the foot is resting on the floor.
   b. For measuring hip flexion, the examinee is in the supine position with both lower extremities and the pelvis stabilized on the table.

Positioning and stabilization of the inclinometer and extender

2. Position the inclinometer and extender (Figure 4-1)
   a. Align the extender of the inclinometer set to the horizontal gravity -0- position with the long axis of the thigh.
   b. The inclinometer should show 0.

Extension of the hip

3. Measuring extension (Figure 4-2)
   a. Establish the neutral -0- starting position for measuring extension in pronation. (See 1a.) Then, ask the examinee to actively lift the lower extremity maximally, keeping the extender aligned with the long axis of the thigh. Read and record the hip extension angle, which actually is a pelvic tilt and lumbar extension (lordosis), as the hip joint does not have anatomical extension.
   b. Ask the examinee to return to the neutral -0- starting position.
   c. Repeat the procedure 2 more times to obtain a valid reading.
   d. Ask the examinee to return to the neutral -0- starting position.

Flexion of the hip

4. Measuring flexion (Figure 4-3)
   a. Establish the neutral -0- starting position for measuring flexion in supination.
   b. See 1b. To stabilize the pelvis, ask the examinee to flex the opposite hip maximally to keep the lumbar spine flat. Ask the examinee to maximally flex the measured hip and when the anterior superior iliac spine (ASIS) start to move, read and record the hip flexion angle.
   c. Ask the examinee to return the hip to the neutral -0- starting position.
   d. Repeat the procedure 2 more times to obtain a valid reading.
   e. Ask the examinee to return to the neutral -0- starting position.

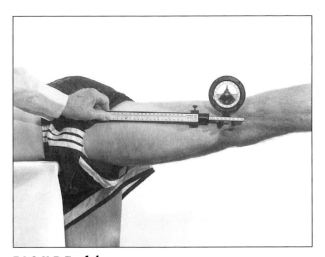

FIGURE 4-1

Neutral -0- starting position of the hip for measuring extension.

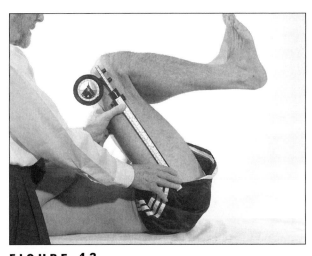

FIGURE 4-3

Measuring flexion of the hip in the supine position.

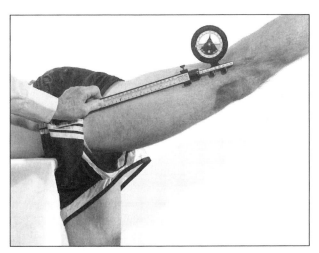

FIGURE 4-2

Measuring extension of the hip.

Validation

5. Validation of rating
   a. The three consecutive measurements should be within 5° of one another or 10% of the mean to be valid.
   b. Use the greatest angle of hip extension and flexion for rating.

Recording

6. Recording
   Record hip extension and flexion and indicate the left or right side.

   Right hip: S: 30 -0- 100

Hip flexion contracture
Extension lag
(restricted motion)

7. Detection of hip flexion contracture (extension lag) (Figure 4-4)
   a. To detect hip flexion contracture, ask the examinee to maximally flex the opposite hip and hold the thigh in this position with both hands (Thomas maneuver). If the measured hip is not in 0 position, measure the contracture (extension lag) angle of the hip with the inclinometer. This angle is the actual starting position and is recorded in the middle of the 3 numbers.

   Right hip: hip flexion contracture
   S: 0-20-100
   (In the above recording, S indicates the sagittal plane, extension is 0, 20° is the actual starting position or extension lag of 20°, and flexion is 100°.)

Measuring in the frontal plane (F)

Abduction and adduction: hip

B. F-Plane: (abduction -0- adduction in 30° flexion)

Neutral -0- starting position:
Examinee position

1. Establish the neutral -0- starting position (Figure 4-5)
   a. To measure hip abduction and adduction with the inclinometer, the examinee has to be placed in the lateral recumbent position on the table (side-lying), so that the frontal plane is vertical.
   b. Ask the examinee to bring the measured extremity into the horizontal position.
   c. Verify it by aligning the extender of the inclinometer, which is set to the horizontal gravity zero position and aligned with the long axis of the thigh. This is the neutral -0- starting position.

Abduction of the hip

2. Measuring abduction (Figure 4-6)
   a. Ask the examinee to maximally abduct the hip (the motion is toward the ceiling). Read and record the hip abduction angle.
   b. Return to the neutral -0- starting position.
   c. Repeat the procedure 2 more times to obtain a valid reading of hip abduction.
   d. Return to the neutral -0- starting position.

Adduction of the hip

3. Preparing for and measuring hip adduction (Figure 4-7)
   a. To measure hip adduction, the measured hip has to be flexed. Use a standardized hip flexion of 30° degrees (similar to shoulder flexion of 30° when measuring adduction of the shoulder).
   b. To measure hip flexion the examinee is asked to roll into the supine position and the hip is flexed 30° (measured with the inclinometer).
   c. The examinee returns to the lateral recumbent position with the measured hip flexed 30°.
   d. Ask the examinee to adduct the measured hip maximally (over the edge of the table with the extender aligned with the long axis of the thigh) then read and record the adduction angle of the hip.

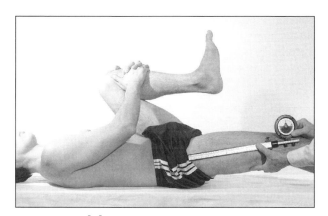

FIGURE 4-4

Measuring hip flexion contracture; extension lag.

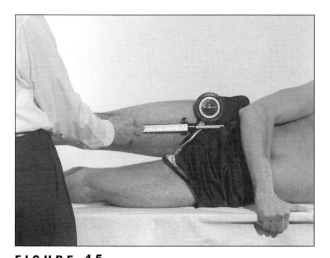

FIGURE 4-5

The hip is in neutral -0- starting position in the frontal plane; side lying.

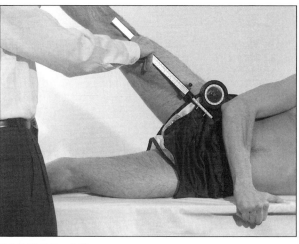

FIGURE 4-6

Measuring hip abduction.

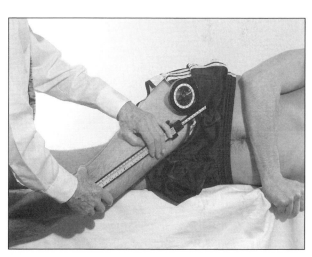

FIGURE 4-7

Measuring hip adduction in 30° of flexion.

e. Return to the neutral -0- starting position.
f. Repeat the procedure 2 more times to obtain a valid reading of hip adduction.
g. Return to the neutral -0- starting position.

Validation

4. Validation of rating
   a. The 3 consecutive measurements should be within 5° of one another or 10% of the mean to be valid.
   b. Use the greatest angle of hip abduction and adduction for rating.

Recording

5. Recording
   Record hip abduction and adduction and record in parentheses the degrees of hip flexion. Indicate the side: left or right.

   Right hip: F: 45 -0- 30 (S 30)

Measuring rotation (R) of the hip

External and internal rotation: hip

C. Measuring rotation: (external rotation -0- internal rotation)

Hip rotation can be measured in 3 ways:

i.) With the hip and knee flexed at 90° and the examinee sitting on the table with the legs hanging over the table edge
ii.) With the hip at 0 and the knee at 90° flexion the examinee is in the prone position on the table with the knee of the examined side flexed 90°
iii.) With the hip and the knee at 0° (stiff knee) the examinee is supine on the table—the long axis of the foot (middle of the heel through the second toe) serves as the indicator of rotation.

To reference the second method (ii.), see *Guides*, Fifth Edition, page 535.

Neutral -0- starting position
Examinee position

1. Establish the neutral -0- starting position
   a. The examinee is in the prone position with the knee of the measured side flexed 90° (the plantar surface of the foot is pointing to the ceiling).

Position and stabilize
the inclinometer and extender

2. Position the inclinometer and extender (Figure 4-8)
   a. The extender with the inclinometer set to the vertical gravity 0 position is aligned with the long axis of the leg (along the tibial crest). The leg is moved (rotated) left or right until it is vertical and the inclinometer shows zero. This is the neutral -0- starting position for hip rotation (mid-position between external and internal rotation).

External rotation of the hip

3. Measuring external rotation (Figure 4-9)
   a. The examinee is asked to fully rotate the hip externally (the foot is moved toward the middle of the body). Read and record the degrees of external rotation.
   b. The examinee returns to the neutral -0- starting position.
   c. The measurement is repeated 2 more times to assure validity.
   d. Return to the neutral -0- starting position.

Internal rotation of the hip

4. Measuring internal rotation
   a. The examinee is asked to fully internally rotate the hip (the foot is moved away from the middle of the body). Read and record the degrees of internal rotation.
   b. The examinee returns to the neutral -0- starting position.

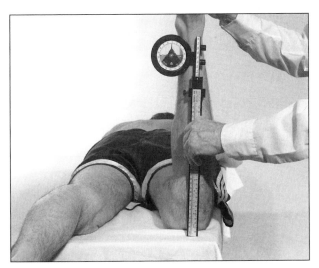

FIGURE 4-8

Neutral -0- starting position for measuring rotation in the prone position.

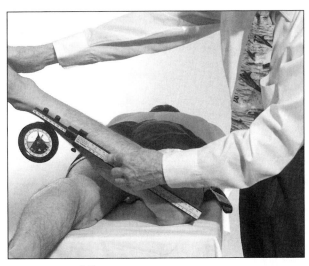

FIGURE 4-9

Measuring external rotation of the hip.

        c. Two more measurements of internal rotation are executed to assure validity.

        d. Return to the neutral -0- starting position.

Validation

5. Validation of rating

        a. The 3 consecutive measurements should be within 5° of one another or 10% of the mean to be valid.

        b. Use the greatest angle of hip external and internal rotation for rating.

Recording

6. Recording

Record external and internal rotation of the hip and state in parentheses the degrees of hip and knee flexion placed behind the initial *R* (for Rotation):

Right hip: R (hip S0, knee S90): 50 -0- 40

ANATOMICAL AREA: KNEE

I. Preparation of Examinee: Refer to Part 1, page 4.

II. Anatomical Landmarks: The long lateral axes of the thigh and the leg, the capitulum fibulae, the lateral malleolus, the long axes of the thigh and the leg in the sagittal plane.

III. Warm-up Exercises: Extend and flex the knee maximally while sitting on the front part of the chair, slowly 4 times. Switch sides and repeat. Also, see Part 1, page 5, exercise numbers 1, 2, 4, 5, 13, 14, and 15.

IV. SFTR Measurements Shown: A. Hyper-extension and flexion B. Valgus/varus is optional in the frontal plane.

Measuring in the sagittal plane (S)

Hyper-extension and flexion of the knee

A. S-Plane: (hyper-extension -0- flexion)

Neutral -0- starting position:
Examinee position

1. Establish the neutral -0- starting position

        a. To measure knee hyper-extension and flexion the examinee is placed in the prone position on the examining table with the feet hanging down beyond the end of the table.

Positioning and stabilization
of the inclinometer and extender

2. Position the inclinometer and extender (Figure 4-10)

        a. The extender with the inclinometer set to horizontal gravity -0- is aligned with the long lateral axis of the leg (parallel to the table) and should indicate 0. If it does not (because the table might not be horizontal), it is set to 0.

        b. The examinee is asked to move the body on the table until the knee is beyond the end of the table. The examiner positions the leg until the inclinometer shows 0. This is the neutral -0- starting position.

Hyper-extension of the knee

3. Measuring hyper-extension (Figure 4-11)

        a. The examiner stabilizes the examinee's thigh on the table and asks the individual to drop the leg toward the floor. If the examinee has hyper-extension (back knee), the examiner reads and records the degree of hyper-extension.

        b. Ask the examinee to return to the neutral -0- starting position.

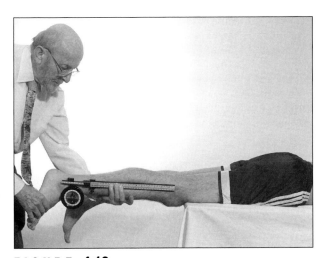

FIGURE 4-10

Neutral -0- starting position of the knee with the knee and leg extending beyond the end of the table.

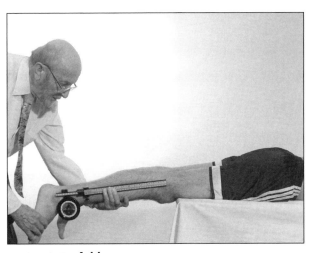

FIGURE 4-11

Measuring hyper-extension of the knee.

c. Repeat this measurement 2 more times to assure validity.

d. Return to the neutral -0- starting position.

Flexion of the knee

4. Measuring flexion (Figure 4-12)

a. The examiner asks the examinee to maximally flex the knee. Then, the examiner reads and records the degrees of flexion.

b. The examinee returns to the neutral -0- starting position.

c. Repeat the measurements 2 more times to validate knee flexion measurements.

d. Have the examinee return to the neutral -0- starting position.

Validation

5. Validation of rating

a. The 3 consecutive measurements should be within 5° of one another or 10% of the mean to be valid.

b. Use the greatest angle of knee extension and flexion for rating.

Recording

6. Recording

Record normal motion of the knee (flexion) in the sagittal plane. Indicate the side: left or right.

Right knee: S: 0 -0- 150

If there is hyper-extension of the knee of 10°, the recording is:

Right knee: S: 10 -0- 150

Note: Flexibility—If there is a problem with tightness of the quadriceps or hamstring muscles, the range of motion of the knee can be measured with the hip flexed at 45°. The hip has to be properly stabilized. See *Guides,* Fifth Edition, page 536, Figure 17-6a.

ANATOMICAL AREA: UPPER ANKLE JOINT, HINDFOOT

I. Preparation of Examinee: Refer to Part 1, page 4.

II. Anatomical Landmarks: The leg: the tibial crest, the long lateral axis of the leg (sagittal plane), the heel, and the plantar side of the long axis of the foot (from the middle of the heel through the second toe). The long axis of the leg (posterior) from the middle of the heel to the middle of the popliteal fossa.

III. Warm-up Exercises: Hold one knee up, extend (dorsiflex) and flex (plantarflex) the foot slowly 4 times. Rotate the ankle clockwise 4 times and counter clockwise 4 times. Change sides and repeat. Also, refer to Part 1, pages 5, 6, exercise numbers 1, 2, 4, 13, 14, 15, and 16.

IV. SFTR Measurements Shown: Ankle extension (dorsiflexion)/flexion (plantar flexion).

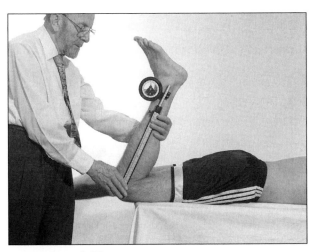

FIGURE 4-12

Measuring flexion of the knee.

Measuring in the sagittal plane (S)

Extension (dorsiflexion) and flexion (plantar flexion): upper ankle joint (hindfoot)

A. S-Plane: (extension -0- flexion)

Neutral -0- starting position
Examinee position

1. Establish the neutral -0- starting position
   a. To measure extension (dorsiflexion) and flexion (plantar flexion) of the foot, have the examinee kneel on a padded chair or examining table with the feet hanging beyond the end of the chair or table. The measured leg is stabilized in the horizontal position. The sole of the foot is vertical in the neutral -0- position.

Positioning and stabilization of the inclinometer and extender

2. Position the inclinometer and extender (Figure 4-13)
   a. The examiner aligns the extender of the inclinometer set to vertical gravity -0- with the long axis of the foot, from the middle of the heel to the second toe and positions the foot until the inclinometer shows 0. This is the neutral starting position.

Extension of the upper ankle joint

3. Measuring extension (Figure 4-14)
   a. The examiner asks the examinee to dorsiflex the foot maximally (the motion is toward the chair) and the degrees of extension are read and recorded.
   b. The examinee returns to the neutral -0- starting position.
   c. Repeat this measurement 2 more times to ensure validity.
   d. Return to the neutral -0- starting position.

Flexion of the upper ankle joint

4. Measuring flexion (Figure 4-15)
   a. The examiner asks the examinee to maximally plantar flex at the ankle. Motion of the sole of the foot is toward the ceiling in the sagittal plane. Read and record the plantar flexion of the upper ankle joint (foot).
   b. Return to the neutral -0- starting position.
   c. Repeat this measurement 2 more times to assure validity.
   d. Return to the neutral -0- starting position.

Validation

5. Validation of rating
   a. The 3 consecutive measurements should be within 5° of one another or 10% of the mean to be valid.
   b. Use the greatest angle of measurement of extension and flexion for rating.

Recording

6. Recording
   Record extension and flexion of the upper ankle joint in the sagittal plane. Indicate side: left or right.

   Left upper ankle joint: S: 20 -0- 40

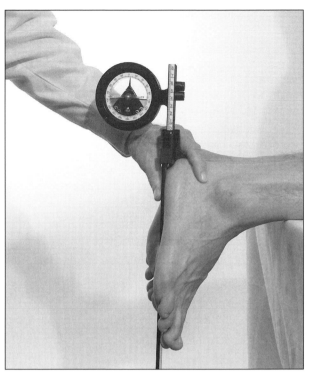

FIGURE 4-13

Neutral -0- starting position of the upper ankle joint in the sagittal plane.

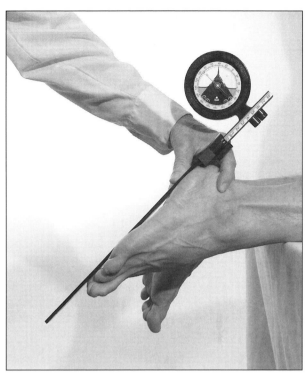

FIGURE 4-15

Measuring flexion (plantar flexion) of the upper ankle joint in the sagittal plane.

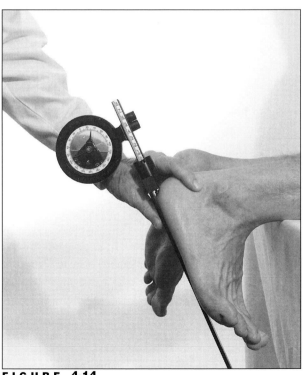

FIGURE 4-14

Measuring extension (dorsiflexion) of the upper ankle joint.

ANATOMICAL AREA: LOWER ANKLE JOINT, HINDFOOT

Definitions of Eversion and Inversion

"Eversion and inversion are very complex movements involving many gliding and rotatory movements between intertarsal and tarsometatarsal joints. As many as 12 different axes of motion have been identified…" [60] Therefore, for practical purposes, eversion and inversion of the hindfoot are measured in the frontal plane, similar to valgus and varus, and recorded as "F." The supination and pronation of the forefoot are measured in a similar way to the supination and pronation of the forearm and recorded as "R," because of predominantly rotatory movements.

I. Preparation of Examinee: Refer to Part 1, page 4.

II. Anatomical Landmarks: The heel, the long axis of the leg posterior (from middle of the heel to the middle of the popliteal fossa), the long axis of the foot, from the middle of the heel to the second toe, the fibula, the tibia, and the calcaneus.

III. Warm-up Exercises: Hold the knee up with both hands, move the ankle up and down 2 times, left and right 2 times, circle clockwise and reverse 4 times. Evert and invert the heel and the foot (out and in) slowly 4 times. See Part 1, pages 5, 6, exercise numbers 1, 2, 4, 13, 14, 15, and 16.

IV. SFTR Measurements Shown: A. Eversion/inversion (valgus/varus)

Measuring in the frontal plane (F)

Eversion and inversion: hindfoot (PPP)*

A. F-Plane: (eversion -0- inversion)

Neutral -0- starting position Examinee position	1. Establish the neutral -0- starting position a. To measure eversion and inversion of the hindfoot, the examinee is in the prone position on the examining table with the knee flexed 90° (the plantar side of the foot toward the ceiling) and the leg is stabilized in this position. The upper ankle joint is in the neutral -0- starting position.
Positioning and stabilization of the inclinometer and extender	2. Position the inclinometer and extender (Figure 4-16) a. Two inclinometers are needed, one to monitor and help keep the leg stabilized in the vertical neutral -0- starting position and the other stabilized over the calcaneus to indicate the degrees of eversion and inversion of the lower ankle joint (subtalar joint). The first inclinometer, which is attached to the extender, is set to the vertical gravity -0- position. The extender is aligned with the long posterior axis of the leg in the frontal plane. The second inclinometer is set to the horizontal gravity -0- position to allow stabilization of the base on the heel in the frontal plane. In neutral -0- starting position, the base of the second inclinometer is perpendicular to the base of the first inclinometer. This is the neutral -0- starting position.

Eversion of the lower ankle joint
(hindfoot)
	3. Measuring eversion (Figure 4-17)
	  a. The examinee is asked to evert the ankle maximally (put the heel into valgus position by moving it away from the middle of the body). The examiner reads and records the deviation (eversion of the hind foot) on the second inclinometer while keeping the first one with the extender and the leg at 0.
	  b. Return the heel to the neutral -0- starting position.
	  c. Repeat this measurement 2 more times to assure validity.
	  d. Return to the neutral -0- starting position.

* PPP=pars posterior pedis

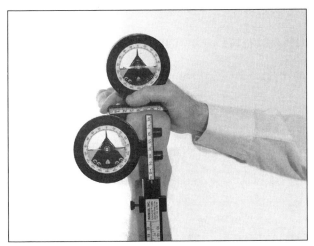

FIGURE 4-16

Neutral -0- starting position of the lower ankle joint in the frontal plane. Two inclinometers are used for measuring eversion and inversion.

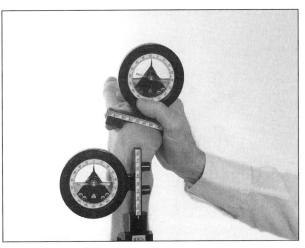

FIGURE 4-17

Measuring eversion of the lower ankle joint; hindfoot and calcaneus valgus.

Inversion of the lower ankle joint (hindfoot)	4. Measuring inversion (Figure 4-18) a. Ask the examinee to invert the ankle (put the heel into varus position by moving it toward the middle of the body). Read and record the inversion angle of the hindfoot. b. Return the foot to the neutral -0- starting position. c. Repeat this measurement 2 more times to assure validity. d. Return to the neutral -0- starting position.
Validation	5. Validation of rating a. The 3 consecutive measurements should be within 5° of one another or 10% of the mean to be valid. b. Use the greatest angle of eversion and inversion for rating.
Recording	6. Recording Record the eversion and inversion of the lower ankle joint (hindfoot) in the frontal plane. Indicate side: left or right. **Right hindfoot: F: 20 -0- 30** **(Lower ankle joint)**

ANATOMICAL AREA: FOREFOOT

I. Preparation of Examinee: Refer to Part 1, page 4.

II. Anatomical Landmarks: The heel, the second toe, the midfoot, the tuberosity of the fifth metatarsal, the metatarsal heads I –V, the fibula, the tibia, and the calcaneus.

III. Warm-up Exercises: Hold the knee up with both hands, move the ankle up and down 2 times, left and right 2 times, circle clockwise 4 times. In addition, see Part 1, pages 5, 6, exercise numbers 1, 2, 4, 13, 14, 15, and 16.

IV. SFTR Measurements Shown: A. Supination/pronation

Measuring rotation (R)

Supination and pronation: forefoot (PAP)

A. Measuring rotation: (supination -0- pronation)

Neutral -0- starting position: Examinee position	1. Establish the neutral -0- starting position The examinee is in the same position as previously, with the knee flexed 90° and the ankle and foot in the neutral -0- starting position.
Positioning and stabilization of the inclinometer	2. Position the inclinometer (Figure 4-19) a. To measure supination and pronation of the forefoot, the starting position is the same, but one inclinometer is stabilized over the midfoot to keep it at zero and the second across the forefoot over the metatarsal heads. b. Both inclinometers are set to horizontal gravity -0- position and show 0 in the neutral -0- starting position.
Supination of the forefoot	3. Measuring supination (Figure 4-20) a. Ask the examinee to supinate the forefoot maximally (move the fibular side of the forefoot toward the ceiling and the planta pedis toward the middle of the body). Read and record the angle of supination. b. Return to the neutral -0- starting position. c. Repeat this measurement 2 more times to assure validity. d. Return to the neutral -0- starting position.

* PAP=pars anterior pedis

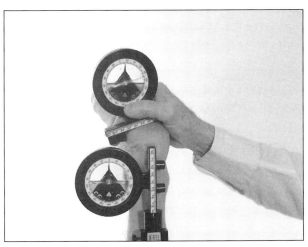

FIGURE 4-18

Measuring inversion of the lower ankle joint, (hindfoot) and calcaneus varus.

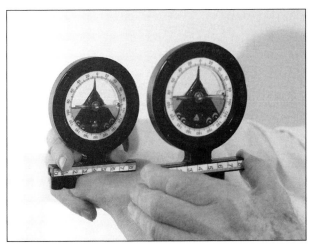

FIGURE 4-19

The forefoot is in neutral -0- starting position. Two inclinometers are used for measuring supination and pronation. Both are set to horizontal gravity -0- position.

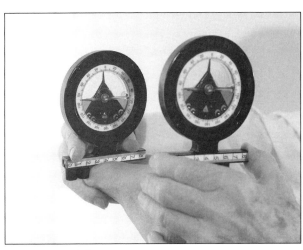

FIGURE 4-20

Measuring forefoot supination.

Pronation of the forefoot

4. Measuring pronation (Figure 4-21)
   a. Ask the examinee to maximally pronate the forefoot (move the tibial side of the forefoot toward the ceiling and the planta pedis away from the middle of the body). Read and record the angle of the forefoot pronation.
   b. Return to the neutral -0- starting position.
   c. Repeat this measurement 2 more times to assure validity.
   d. Return to the neutral -0- starting position.

Validation

5. Validation of rating
   a. The 3 consecutive measurements should be within 5° of one another or 10% of the mean to be valid.
   b. Use the greatest angle of supination and pronation of the forefoot for rating.

Recording

6. Recording
   Record supination and pronation of the forefoot as rotation (R). Indicate the side: left or right.

   Right forefoot: R: 30 -0- 20

ANATOMICAL AREA: TOES

Stabilization Devices

To measure the range of motion of the toes, a ¼ inch plate or a hand stabilization device is needed. (These may be the same tools as those used when measuring the thumb and fingers.) A chair may be placed at the side and close to the end of the examining table. The stabilization plate is set on the chair with the margin of the plate protruding 2 to 3 inches beyond the edge of the chair.

Measurement of the toes is done similarly to measurement of the fingers of the hand. Extension and flexion are measured in the sagittal plane and abduction and adduction in the transverse plane.

Note: The big toe has 2 functional units: the metatarsophalangeal joint (MTP I) and the interphalangeal joint (IPH). The toes have three functional units: the MTP joints II-V, the proximal interphalangeal joints (PIP) II-V, and the distal interphalangeal joints (DIP) II-V.

ANATOMICAL AREA: THE BIG TOE METATARSOPHALANGEAL JOINT (MTP I)

I. Preparation of Examinee: Refer to Part 1, page 4.

II. Anatomical Landmarks: Identify the toes and their joints, the long axes of metatarsals II-V, and the toes (digits I-V).

III. Warm-up Exercises: Hold the knee up with both hands, move the ankle up and down 2 times, left and right 2 times, circle clockwise and reverse 4 times. Also, dorsiflex (extend) and flex (curl) the toe 8 times. In addition, see Part 1, pages 5, 6, exercise numbers 1, 2, 4, 13, 14, 15, and 16.

IV. SFTR Measurements Shown: A. Extension/flexion B. Abduction (valgus) and adduction (varus) are optional.

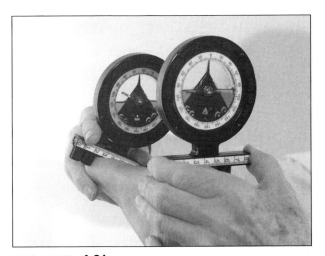

FIGURE 4-21

Measuring forefoot pronation.

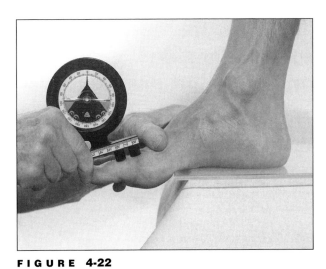

FIGURE 4-22

Neutral -0- starting position of the metatarsophalangeal joint of the big toe (MTP I) in the sagittal plane. The foot is stabilized on the stabilization plate, which is placed on a chair. The examinee is sitting on an examination table.

Measuring in the sagittal plane (S)

Extension and flexion: big toe

A. S-Plane: (extension -0- flexion)

The examinee is sitting on the table with one leg hanging down at the end of the table. The foot of the measured side is placed on the 1/4-inch stabilization plate on a chair with the knee flexed about 90° and the foot in neutral -0- starting position.

Neutral -0- starting position: Examinee position

1. Establish the neutral -0- starting position
   a. The foot including the big toe to be measured is placed on the stabilization plate or the hand stabilization device.

Positioning and stabilization of the inclinometer

2. Position the inclinometer (Figure 4-22)
   a. The inclinometer, set to horizontal gravity -0- position, is stabilized on the proximal phalanx of the big toe and set to 0, if 0 is not already indicated.
   b. The examinee is asked to move the foot forward so that the MTP I joint is beyond the margin of the plate and can move freely.
   c. The examinee positions the proximal phalanx so that the inclinometer shows 0. This is the neutral -0- starting position.
   d. The metatarsal I is stabilized on the plate or stabilization device by holding it down.

Extension of the MTP I

3. Measuring extension (Figure 4-23)
   a. Ask the examinee to extend the big toe maximally (the motion is toward the ceiling). Measure and record the extension in the MTP I joint.
   b. Have the examinee return to the neutral -0- starting position.
   c. Repeat this measurement 2 more times to assure validity.
   d. Have the examinee return to the neutral -0- starting position.

Flexion of the MTP I

4. Measuring flexion (Figure 4-24)
   a. Ask the examinee to maximally flex the big toe in the MTP I joint. Read and record the angle of flexion in the MTP I joint.
   b. Have the examinee return to the neutral -0- starting position.
   c. Repeat this measurement 2 more times to assure validity.
   d. Have the examinee return to the neutral -0- starting position.

Validation

5. Validation of rating
   a. The 3 consecutive measurements should be within 5° of one another or 10% of the mean to be valid.
   b. Use the greatest angle of extension and flexion for rating.

Recording

6. Recording
   Record extension and flexion of the big toe in the MTP I joint of the big toe. Indicate side: left or right.

   Right big toe: MTP I; S: 50 -0- 30

   Neutral -0- starting position of the IPH is shown (Figure 4-25).

   Proceed similarly to measure flexion in the IPH joint (Figure 4-26). Recording is:

   Right big toe: IPH; S: 0 -0- 30

   (Normally, there is no extension.)

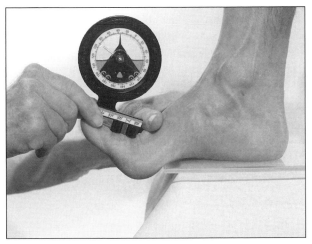

FIGURE 4-23

Measuring extension (dorsiflexion) of the metatarsophalangeal joint of the big toe (MTP I) in the sagittal plane.

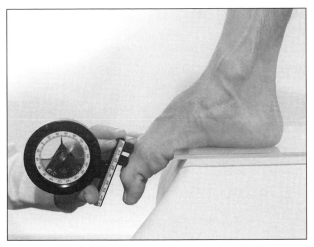

FIGURE 4-24

Measuring flexion (plantar flexion) of the metatarsophalangeal joint of the big toe (MTP I) in the sagittal plane.

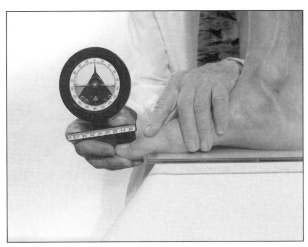

FIGURE 4-25

Neutral -0- starting position of the interphalangeal joint of the big toe (IPH).

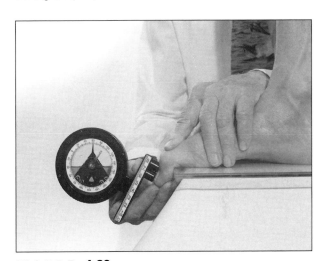

FIGURE 4-26

Measuring flexion of the interphalangeal joint of the big toe (IPH).

ANATOMICAL AREA: TOES II THROUGH V

The toes II through V are measured in a similar fashion. Indicate side: left or right. The recordings in the metatarsophalangeal joint are:

40° extension and 30° flexion, left second toe:

Left MTP II: S: 40 -0- 30

30° extension and 20° flexion in the MTP joint of the third right toe:

Right MTP III: S: 30 -0- 20

20° extension and 10° flexion in the MTP joint of the left fourth toe:

Left MTP IV: S: 20 -0- 10

10° extension and 10° flexion in the MTP joint of the right little toe:

Right MTP V: S: 10 -0- 10